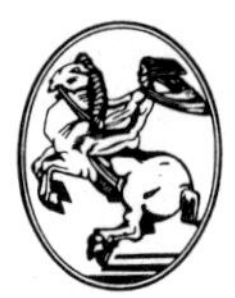

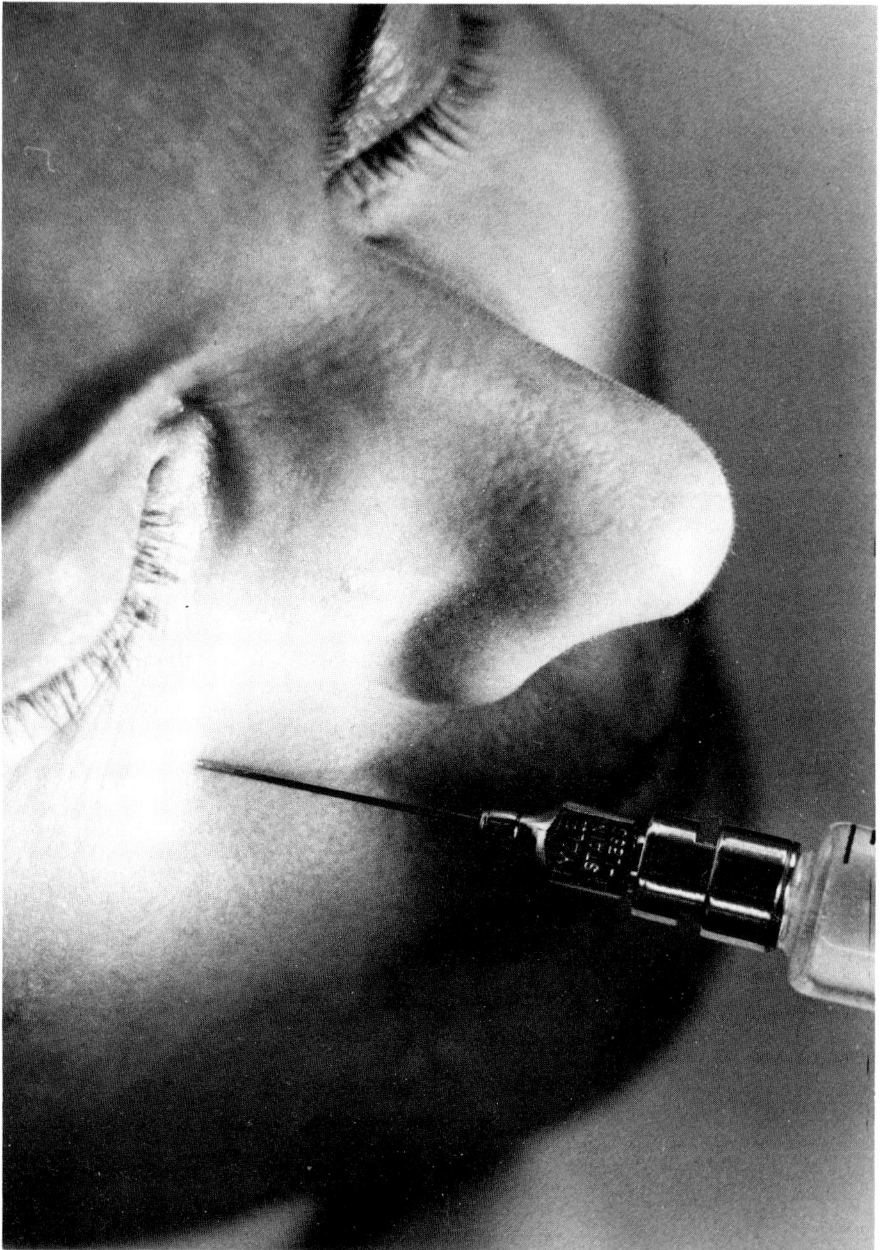

Peripheral Nerve Block

Pharmacologic – By Local Anesthesia
Electric – By Transdermal Stimulation

F. L. Jenkner

Springer-Verlag
Wien New York

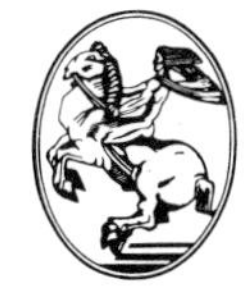

Fritz Lothar Jenkner, M.D., F.I.C.S., F.N.Y.C.S.
Associate Professor of surgery/neurosurgery
University of Vienna Medical School
Consultant for pain problems
The Ludwig Boltzmann Institute for Clinical Oncology
Head, Pain Clinic at the Out Patient Institution, Vienna

Revised and enlarged translation of the 2nd German edition
of "Nervenblockaden – Indikationen und Technik"
Wien – New York: Springer-Verlag 1975

Translated by the author and Ute Jenkner, M. A., Ph. D., Vienna

With 72 Figures
Drawings by M. Stelzel, Vienna

Printed in Austria by Ferd. Berger & Söhne OHG, A-3580 Horn, NÖ.

Library of Congress Cataloging in Publication Data. Jenkner, Fritz L. Peripheral nerve block. Translation of Nervenblockaden. Bibliography: p. 1. Nerve block. I. Title. RD84.J4313 617.966 77-8317

ISBN 3-211–81426-4 Springer-Verlag Wien – New York
ISBN 0-387-81426-4 Springer-Verlag New York – Wien
ISBN 3-211-81290-3 2. deutsche Auflage
Springer-Verlag Wien – New York
ISBN 0-387-81290-3 2nd German edition
Springer-Verlag New York – Wien

Introduction

Fifty years ago surgeons often performed various operations in conduction anesthesia or local anesthesia in the hope of circumventing pulmonary complications. The preparation for the operation was the task of an assistant who had to know and carry out the diverse local anesthetic procedures and who was responsible for their effectiveness. In this way a large number of physicians learned to carry out nerve blocks, which they also applied more and more outside their operative duties.

The introduction of modern general anesthesia led almost to the disappearance of the special techniques of nerve blocking at the former "classic" places of their teaching. Therefore it is a great merit of my former associate F. L. Jenkner to recall the art of nerve blocking, be it for diagnostic or therapeutic purposes. He presents the many possibilities as an addition to the therapeutic armamentarium and explains their indications, bases, and techniques.

I do not think that one needs to be a specialist to carry out these useful techniques; but one has to have an understanding of certain topographic-anatomic situations, and one needs to know the rules of the procedure to obviate the risks that are always inherent in any disruption of the integrity of the integument of the human body. Thus by presenting all the mentioned aspects a renaissance of good though old practices may be initiated in the light of new achievements.

F. Spath
Professor emeritus,
Department of Surgery
University of Graz,
Graz, Austria

Preface

An understanding of the perception of pain impulses and of their conduction and processing to the sensation of pain provides the basis for what is generally called treatment of painful conditions. The most rational method of this therapy is to remove the causes of pain, i. e., of the noxious agents or conditions leading to pain. This, however, is not always possible. Therefore methods of interruption of pain conduction (so-called conduction anesthesia or nerve blocking) are gaining importance. Destructive surgical approaches for lasting interruption of conduction pathways or dorsal column stimulation by implanted electrodes should be considered only as a last resort. A third approach is the modification of personal engagement in pain perception, which may be achieved by either psychotherapy, psychopharmacological agents, or psychosurgery. The method most commonly applied for relieving pain is the use of analgesics that raise the threshold of pain.

Regional anesthesia came into being in 1848 when Koller demonstrated the effect of cocaine to ophthalmologists. Infiltration then became possible by the invention of the injection needle by Alexander Wood (1853). Difficult problems of general or regional measures for the treatment of pain should be handled by anesthetists. However, conditions of pain that allow one to obtain a painless state by nerve blocking are so frequent that other physicians are frequently confronted by them. Specialists in internal medicine, surgery, orthopedics, as well as general practitioners – with some dexterity – may easily achieve proficiency in a number of simple blocking procedures, which they may use to the benefit of their patients.

The present work began as notes to a lecture series. It is hoped that it will inform interested physicians about indications, techniques, evaluation of effects, possible complications, dosages, and kinds of local anesthetics as well as the duration of some of the more frequently used nerve blocks by means of sketches and concise discussions.

This material is presented in such a way as to allow the reader to obtain a maximum of information in a minimum of time. The excellent responses, mainly from general practitioners, prompted the presentation of this monograph in the English language, as suggested by Springer-Verlag New York. In this edition a small chapter on transdermal stimulation has been added, because this most modern method promises to become of great importance in the relief of pain.

F. L. Jenkner

Vienna, 1977

Contents

Transdermal Stimulation 103

General Section

Application of Nerve Blocks

In spite of the great strides made by general anesthesia to date, conduction anesthesia has gained increasing importance in temporary relief of pain itself as well as in enabling surgeons to carry out some minor procedures that must be done immediately or are performed more easily this way (e. g., in cases of dislocated shoulder). If blocking a nerve is accompanied by positive effects on other organs, thereby improving the condition of a patient (e. g., spreading of solution to stellate ganglion in brachial plexus block and thereby possibly improving an existing hypoxic cardiac state), it is preferred to a general anesthetic. If metabolic disorders are present (such as diabetes), routine intubation anesthesia carries a certain risk. Such risks may not exist if the (simple) required procedure is carried out under a nerve block. It should, however, be recalled that nerve blocking should not be performed in children under about 10 to 12 years of age. Also neurasthenics, neurotics, and depressive patients (these latter presenting possible symptoms of organic diseases as signs of their psychic disorder) do not allow one to expect good results from therapeutic blocks. The majority of pathologic states that may be ameliorated by nerve blocking are presented together with the respective blocking procedure. Some indications are not generally accepted but are included because of the experience of the author. One basic principle is imperative and generally accepted: Only the smallest amount of anesthetic in a solution of the lowest possible concentration of which a certain effect is to be expected should be used.

Premedication

Some practitioners always use premedication. This author, however, is of the opinion that normal adults do not require any premedication for diagnostic, prognostic, or therapeutic blocking. All drugs used for premedication (such as nembutal, dilantin, lytic cocktail, or the like) are apt to narrow the sensorium of a patient to such an extent that they prevent an exact verbalization of paresthesias or tingling sensations by the patient, thereby masking the immediate effect of a blockade. Only with nerve blocking for surgical procedures is premedication (including atropine) advised. Even here, patients in shock do not require premedication. If children have to be blocked, they should be premedicated. Geriatric patients may be given small doses of a mild neuroleptic, but in general they also do not require premedication at all. A so-called light premedication is not at all recommended. Instead, it should be stated that careful psychologic handling of the patient and cultivation of a good patient-doctor relationship always renders premedication unnecessary.

Mode of Action of Local Anesthetics

Understanding the action of local anesthetics as means for interruption of nerve conduction needs only a brief and very fragmentary knowledge of physiology and pharmacology. Those more interested in the problem are referred to the extensive literature on the subject. Here, only the essentials will be sketched briefly.

The subjective sensation of pain is possible only with a conscious subject and with intact conduction pathways from the (adequate) stimulus in the periphery to the central organ, i. e., the brain. Every interruption of these pathways, wherever it occurs, prevents the sensation of pain. The effect of local anesthetics consists in a temporary interruption of these pathways. The time limit of the effect gives the duration of the effect, whereas the interval from application (= injection) to the beginning of the effect constitutes the time of onset (or latency).

All local anesthetics are available as aqueous solutions of their salts. They must be carried to the nerves by extracellular fluids and therefore they must have a hydrophilic group. On the other hand, they need to be fat soluble to enter a nerve, which means that they must also have a lipophilic group in their structure. Consequently, local anesthetics have in principle the following chemical structure:

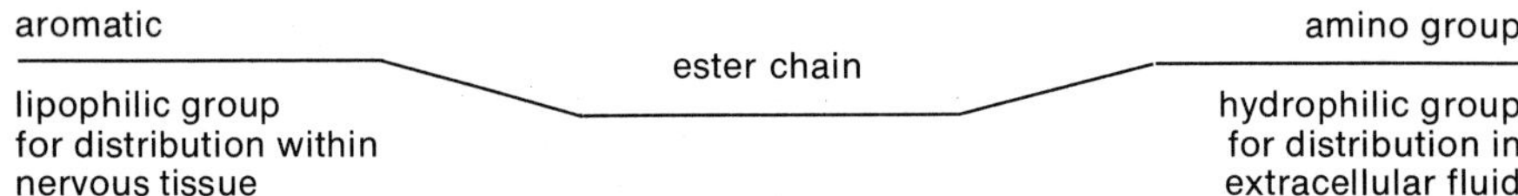

From the salts, tissue alkali liberates the free base which enters the nerve cell and stabilizes its membrane to potassium loss; the nerve remains in a state of rest, i. e., polarized. Depolarization, a characteristic feature of nerve conduction, may not occur. Sodium chloride and carbon dioxide are the two other substances split off the salt by tissue alkali. The more acid a salt is, the faster the base is liberated. Lengthening the ester chain lowers basicity, lowers solubility, and increases toxicity and relative potency.

Schematic of membrane potentials

```
- - - + + + + + + + + + + + +        - - - + + + + + + + + + + + +
+ + + - - - - - - - - - - - -        + + + - - - - - - - - - - - -

+ + + + + + - - - + + + + + +        - - - + + + + + + + + + + + +
- - - - - - + + + - - - - - -        + + + - - - - - - - - - - - -

+ + + + + + + + + + + + - - -        - - - + + + + + + + + + + + +
- - - - - - - - - - - - + + +        + + + - - - - - - - - - - - -
```

In conduction — In interruption of conduction

Onset and duration of the interruption of conduction depends on the time required for the local anesthetic to penetrate all fibers of a given nerve. Small fibers will be interrupted sooner than larger ones. Therefore nerves conducting vasospastic impulses will be interrupted almost immediately, followed by those conducting pain impulses. Then sensory and last motor fibers are interrupted. It may be mentioned that this sequence of events is just the reverse of the sequence in the event of pressure on a nerve: Here motor fibers suffer first, followed by sensation, pain, and vasomotricity.
To influence pain, the blocking of a nerve must be carried out between the stimulus producing pain and the central site of processing to the conscious sensation of pain. This means that, in the case of projected pain, the site of stimulation (e. g., an intervertebral foramen) must be found; only if the block is carried out central to this location will the pain disappear. Any procedure at a place peripheral to the stimulus is absolutely ineffective.

Choosing the Anesthetic

There is available a whole series of local anesthetics, a small selection of which is given in the table on page 6. However large this number seems, one may safely limit the application of these to only two or three out of the selection of four given below. These are described with all the details necessary for their proper use. Properties required for optimal effects are fast onset, great depth, good penetration, long duration of action, total reversibility, and no tissue toxicity. There should also exist good chemical stability. All these properties usually are compared to procaine, which is given the therapeutic potency and toxicity of 1 simply because from 1907 to 1947 no other local anesthetic could compare with it. This historic reason is the only one for citing it here, because today, procaine should never be used for nerve blocking.

Procaine hydrochloride (Novocaine) was synthesized in 1907 and was the leading local anesthetic up to 1947; the maximum single dose without adrenaline is 500 mg (with adrenaline it is 1000 mg). Duration of action is 45 min, beginning 5 to 10 min after injection. Partially because of this short action, but more because it is an ester and immediately upon injection is split by esterases (which are always present in blood and tissues) and one of the split products is *para*-aminobenzoic acid, an allergene, it is not wise to use it for nerve blocking.

Lidocaine hydrochloride (Xylocaine, Lignocaine) was synthesized in 1943 by Löfgren. The pH of a 2 percent solution is 6.9. Lidocaine diffuses into tissue four times better than procaine. Its toxicity is 2, its potency is 4; its cumulative toxicity is 6 mg/kp of body weight. The maximum single dose without adrenaline is 200 mg, with adrenaline it is 400 mg. A 0.8 percent solution suffices for synaptic blocking of sympathetic fibers; for analgesia a 1 percent solution and for muscular relaxation a 2 percent solution is required. Duration of action without adrenaline: 2 percent, 60 min; 1 percent, 50 min; with adrenaline: 2 percent, 135 min; 1 percent, 80 min; latency 2 min.

Mepivacaine hydrochloride (Carbocaine) was synthesized 1953 by Ekenstam. The pH of a 2 percent solution is 6.8 to 6.9. Toxicity without adrenaline is 1.5 to 2; with adrenaline it is 0.5. Its cumulative toxicity is 8 mg/kp of body weight. Its potency is 4. The maximum single dose without (with) adrenaline is 300 (500) mg. Duration of action without (with) adrenaline at 2 percent is 100 (135) min, at 1 percent is 70 (90) min. It has greater affinity to nervous tissue than lidocaine. It has no vasodilatatory property and therefore is resorbed much more slowly; it is to be preferred where adrenaline is contraindicated, as in geriatric patients. Its latency is somewhat shorter than lidocaine (37). Duration of action without adrenaline is 40 percent longer than lidocaine, with adrenaline it equals that of lidocaine.

Prilocaine hydrochloride (Xylonest) was synthesized in 1960 by Wielding. The pH of a 2 percent solution is 4.6. Its toxicitiy is 1.5 to 4, its potency is 4. The maximum single dose without adrenaline is 400 mg; with adrenaline it is 600 mg. Cumulative toxicity is 7 mg/kp of body weight, but may lead to methemoglobinemia. For muscular relaxation a 2 percent solution is required. Duration and latency is as for lidocaine. It has less vasodilatatory effect than lidocaine, in this respect more resembling mepivacine. The addition of adrenaline only barely prolongs the action. It is contraindicated in cases of insufficient O_2 levels in the blood.

Bupivacaine hydrochloride (Marcaine) was synthesized in 1947 by Ekenstam. The pH of a 0.5 percent solution is 6.3 to 6.6. Its toxicity is 8, its potency is 16. It is less cumulating than lidocaine or mepivacaine. The maximum single dose without (with) adrenaline is 150 mg (2.5 mg/kg body weight within 3 hr). Analgesia is obtained with a 0.25 percent solution, muscular relaxation with a 0.5 percent solution. Duration of action without (with) adrenaline at 0.5 percent is 300 (400) min; at 0.25 percent it is 200 (300) min. With adrenaline, the 0.5 percent solution may have a duration of up to 1500 min and longer, if the area injected is not very vascular. On the average, duration is three times longer and twice as deep as with mepivacaine. This substance represents a true improvement for anesthetists looking for an extremely long acting local anesthetic.

Note: Data on kind and quantity of local anesthetic to be used for a certain blocking procedure should be regarded under the criteria of the substances just given. It is not possible to mention all drugs with every nerve block. The physician carrying out the procedure will have to make his selection accordingly. One should, however, recall that solutions of higher concentration are resorbed faster than equal amounts of a drug as a weaker solution. Therefore, the single maximum doses given are for average concentrations; in lower concentrations, they may be up to 25 percent higher, in the highest concentrations up to 20 percent less. When using various concentrations this should be remembered. If a block is used for a diagnostic procedure, a very short-acting and fast-acting drug is preferable. For therapeutic blocks, long-acting local anesthetics should be preferred.
Local anesthetics should be used in the form of ampoules only on which name and batch number are imprinted. This is to assure errors from, for example, injecting al-

Comparison of Several Local Anesthetics

Generic name	Proprietary name	Relative analgesic potency	Relative toxicity	Single maximum dose in mg without adrenaline (adult, 70 kp)	Single maximum dose in mg with adrenaline (adult, 70 kp)	Type	Time for onset in min	duration with adrenaline	duration without adrenaline	Vasodilatation
Procaine	Novocaine	1	1	500	1.000	E	5–10	–45	60	Yes
Tetracaine	Pantocaine	10–15	10	20	100	E	10	60	–90	Yes
Lidocaine	Xylocaine	4	2	200	500	A	–2	60	–180	Yes
Prilocaine	Xylonest	4	1,5	400	600	A	–2	60	–120	Some
Mepivacaine	Carbocaine	4	2	300	500	A	1	100	–180	No
Bupivacaine	Marcaine	10	4	150		A	2–5	300	–900	No
Butanilicaine	Hostacaine	4	2	*)	*)	A	–2	60	–150	Yes
Tolycaine	Baycaine	*)	*)	250	600	E+A	2–5	60	–90	Yes

E = **ester:** In solution of limited stability, procaine has limited capacity for penetration. It is split by (most probably) pseudocholinesterase in *p*-aminobenzoic acid, which acts as an allergene and may cause sensitization. The latter causes allergic side effects, which are known for this type of local anesthetic.
A = **amide type:** Allergic reactions are unknown for this type of local anesthetic. They are not split in tissue nor are they metabolized in the liver. Single maximum dose is given for normal pharmacokinesis and excretory conditions. Therefore, in case of severe renal insufficiency and liver damage these drugs should not be given in full single maximum dose.
*) No data.

cohol instead of local anesthetic. This does not apply only to use in an office procedure. Today all needles and syringes should be used only once and then discarded. In this way sharpness of needles and cleanliness and sterility are assured and the possibility of provoking hepatitis is obviated. Unfortunately, for some blocks longer needles than those available in disposable packs are required. 3.6 and 8 cm needles do not cause a problem. It is at 10, 12, and 15 cm that it is still necessary to clean and resterilize needles. For practical purposes it is advised that after sterilization each needle be put in a separate vial with the point in a cotton pellet at the bottom of the vial. The sterile vial is then closed by a stopper. After use, the unsterile needle is inserted into the vial the other way around to distinguish clearly sterile from used needles.

Additions to Local Anesthetics

With the exception of mepivacaine and bupivacaine, all local anesthetic substances have a more or less vasoconstricting property. Therefore the action is not so very long and lends itself to prolongation by various additions. This has been done for a long time.

In general, vasoconstricting agents are used for the purpose. We prefer not to use vasoconstricting agents not only because adrenaline is apt to cause undue side effects, but also because such agents may affect a patient's blood pressure in an adverse manner. This statement is stressed in spite of the fact that relevant ready mixtures are available commercially. If one desires to use these mixtures, as ear, nose and throat specialists usually do, an optimal concentration of adrenaline is 1:200,000 in the solution; higher concentrations do not increase vasoconstriction or prolong time of action, but only increase undesirable side effects. Where adrenaline causes sensitivity reactions, *n*-adrenaline may be preferred, which almost never has such actions.

Other possibilities for prolonging the action of a local anesthetic twice to fivefold is to admix an equal amount of "periston N," a substance with very high molecular weight, to the solution with higest concentration (lidocaine 2 percent, bupivacaine 0.5 percent). This mixture, however, is not available commercially and should be prepared just prior to injection. Its components are available commercially, and this combination has found relatively wide application. Prolongation of action to several weeks or longer is obtained by admixing ammonia sulfate (20 percent solution) with equal parts of a local anesthetic in high concentration. This most effective mixture then contains half the concentration of the local anesthetic and 10 percent ammonia sulfate. It is said to have a duration of action of up to 4 to 6 weeks. Others, however, have been unable to duplicate this observation. Side effects, as seen with phenol or 96 percent alcohol, in the form of necroses have not been reported with the ammonia sulfate mixture. However, because the 20% solution of ammonia sulfate has to be prepared magistraliter, the mixture has not gained wide acceptance.

Pain Conduction and Pain Projection

The projection of the subjective sensation of pain originating in an organ, is quite specific for that organ and is directed to a specific area of the body: One speaks of pain projection. Knowledge of this projection is certainly reflected in the experience of older physicians, and is frequently spoken of as "clinical vision." However, knowledge about the correlation of somato-segmentary innervation of organs as well as autonomic (sympathetic) correlation of segmental nature to these organs or vessels is most essential for the achievement of therapeutic effects via blocking the respective somatic or sympathetic nerves.

There follows a tabular survey correlating some of the more important organs and their somatic and sympathetic segmentary innervations. This table is not intended to be complete; but it represents an attempt to provide assistance to the less experienced with hints to those segments the blocking of which may give good results in relieving pain or other conditions amenable by nerve blocks.

Naturally, projection of pain is a much more complicated process than can be indicated here. In addition to the primary region where pain originates, the specific area to which pain is projected from the primary area is just as important for the patient and just as distressing or characteristic, as these characteristics of pain projection are an important indication for the experienced pointing to the painful organ or area of body.

The table presented, however, should not seduce one to simply relieve all pain in a certain region by nerve blocking and forget about the basic process underlying the pain. It should rather help to bridge the time gap between finding the reasons for pain and the beginning of rational therapy by definite measures when these are possible. Or it should help to alleviate pain by multiple blocks of nerves in those unfortunate patients suffering from malignancies that are no longer operable or that are no longer amenable to treatment. This last use is especially common in some countries and is gaining reputation in others. In these cases nerve blocking combines relief of pain of sometimes long duration with preservation of mental power and undisturbed sensorium (quite contrary to the action of narcotics, which are being used much too frequently and freely). Blocks may be repeated several times, and in these cases should be given interchangeably as somatic and sympathetic blocks of the respective segments. This is because not all pain is mediated via somatic nerves but vascular pain impulses sometimes originate in vascular spasticity and the latter is positively influenced by sympathetic blocking. These alternative blockades have gained much favor in treatment of pain of malignancy.

In giving segmentary correlation of various organs, it should be noted that various authors have divergent opinions, especially concerning autonomic (sympathetic) fibers. The range presented here coincides with the segments agreed upon by most authors. If one disregards the extreme segments, given in brackets, and adheres to blocking the median of the given segments, positive results of the interruption of pathways may certainly be expected. If the epidural segmental approach is used, the spread of solution should also be calculated to give interruption in additional segments next to the one injected.

Survey of Pain Projection

	Organ	Pain projection	Pain conduction via segmental nerves	Origin of preganglionic sympatic fibers	
Head and neck	Meninges	Scalp	Nucl. sens. N. V.* IX, X u. XII	Th 1–Th 2 (3)	via stellate ganglion
	Eye	Eye socket and forehead	Nucl. sens. N. V. (first branch)	Th 1– Th 3 (4)	
	Tear glands	Eye socket	Nucl. tract. solit. N. VII u. IX	Th 1, Th 2	
	Parotid gland	Parotid region	Nucl. tract. solit. N. V via N. VII + IX	Th 1, Th 2	
	Salivatory glands	Submandibular region	Nucl. tract. solit., N. ling. via N. VII and geniculate ganglion	Th 1, Th 2	
	Thyroid gland	Ventral part of neck	C 2–C 4 Th 1, Th 2	Th 1, Th 2	
	Larynx	Throat and ventral part of neck	N. laryng. sup. ganglion	Th 2–Th 7	
Thorax	Trachea, bronchi	About the sternum	Th2–Th 7	Th 2–Th 7	
	Lung parenchyma	Insensitive for pain	Insensitive for pain	Th 2–Th 7	
	Parietal pleura in area of: Shoulder	Shoulder	C 3–C 5		
	Supraclavicular	Supraclavicular (brachial plexus)	C 8–Th 1		
	Intercostal	Intercostal nerves	Th 1uTh 12		
	Heart	Precordium and left (right) arm	Th 1–Th 4 (5)	Th 1–Th 4 (5)	
	Thoracic aorta	Upper half of thorax and neck	Th 1–Th 5 (6)	Th 1uTh 5	
	Abdominal aorta	Lower half of thorax and abdomen	Th 6uTh 12	Th 6–L 2	
	Esophagus Upper half Lower half	Mid-sternum	Th 5–Th 8	Th 2–Th 5 Th 5–Th 8	

* Roman numerals refer to cranial nerves.

	Stomach	Epigastric and interscapular region	Th (6) 7, Th 8 (9)	Th (5) 6–Th 10 (11)
	Liver and gall bladder	Right hypochondrium	Th (5) 6–Th 8 (9) and phrenic nerve	Th 6–Th 11 right
	Pancreas	Epigastrium, lower part of sternum, midline on back in area of 10th and 11th rib	Th (5) 6–Th 10 (11) and vagus nerve celiac ganglion	Th 5–Th 11 left
	Spleen	Left hypogastric area	Th 6–Th 8	Th 6–Th 8
	Small intestine:			
	Duodenum	Epigastrium and	Th (5) 6–Th 7 (8*)	Th 6–Th 11
	Jejunum and ileum	Umbilical area	Th 9–Th 11	
	Large intestine:			
	Cecum and ascending colon	Suprapubic area	Th 9–Th 11	Th 8–Th 11 right
	Appendix	Right lower quadrant	Th 10–Th 11 (–L 1)	Th 8–Th 11 right
Abdomen	Descending colon and sigma	Deep pelvic area and anus	L 1 and L 2 S 2–S 4	Th 11–Th 12 L 1–L 4 left
	Adrenal gland	None	None	Th 6–L 2 unilateral
	Kidney	Hip and groin	Th 10–L 2	Th 10–L 1 (2) unilateral
	Ureter	From back to groin	Th 11–L 2	Th 11–L 1 (2) unilateral
	Urinary bladder:			
	Fundus	Suprapubic area	Th 11–L 1	L 1–L 2 (hypogastric nerve)
	Neck	Perineal and anal region	S 2–S 4	
	Testicles	Testes	Th 10	Th 10–L 1
	Prostate gland	Perineal area and lower back	Th 10, Th 11 S 2–S 4	Th 10–L 1
	Ovaries and tubes	Both lower quadrants	Th 10	Th 6–L 2
	Uterus	Perineum, lower pelvic area	Th 10–L 1, S 2–S 4	Th 6–L 2
	Female external genitalia	Perineum and local	S 2–S 4	L 1–L 2
Extremities	Blood vessels, sweat glands, hair follicles etc. of:			
	Upper extremity	Local on skin	C 5–Th 1	Th 2–Th 8 (9)
	Trunk	Local on skin	Th 1–Th 12	Th 1–Th 12
	Lower extremity	Local an skin	L 4–S 3	Th 10–L 3

* Oral half right, aboral half left and vagus nerve.

This table on pain projection is supplemented by data on segmental (radicular) nerve supply of some of the more important muscles and reflexes.

Segmental Correspondence of Muscles

Deep muscles of neck	C 1–4	Intercostals	D 1–12
Sternocleidomastoid	C 1–3	Abdominals	D 6–12
Trapezius muscle	C 2–4	Iliopsoas	L 1–4
Diaphragm	C 3–5	Gluteus maximus	L 5–S 2
Pectoralis muscle	C 5–8, D 1	Gluteus medius	L 4–S 1
Deltoid muscle	C 5–6	Quadriceps and abductors	L 2–4
Biceps, brachioradialis	C 5–6	Biceps, semimembranaceus and semitendinosus	L 5–S 2
Triceps muscle	C 6–8	Soleus, gastrocnemius	L 5–S 2 (3)
Extendors of wrist and fingers	C (5) 6-7 (8)	Peroneal group	L 5–S 1 (2)
Flexors of wrist and fingers	C 7–D 1	Perineal and sphincters	S 3–5

Segmental Correspondence of Reflexes

Deep (tendon) reflexes:		Superficial reflexes:	
Jaw jerk	trigeminal	Ciliospinal	C 8–D 1
Biceps	C 5–6	Epigastric	D 7–8
Triceps	C 6–7	Upper abdominal	D 8–9
Wrist	C 8–D 1	Lower abdominal	D 10–11
Knee	L 2–4	Suprapubic	D 12
Ankle	S 1 + 2	Cremasteric	L 1 + 2
		Gluteal	L 4–5
		Plantar	S 1–2
		Anal reflex	S 5

Sclerotomes on Arm and Leg

In addition to this segmental survey, presentation of sclerotomes of arm and leg (from V. T. Inman and J. B. de C. M. Saunders, Referred pain from skeletal structures, J. Nerv. Ment. Dis. *99:* 660, 1944) helps to recognize those segments (figures on pages 12 and 13) or nerves (figures on pages 14 and 15) responsible for conduction of pain impulses from various skeletal structures to our consciousness. This is not only important for treating articular pain but also essential for abolishing pain from malignant bone lesions (primary or secondary).

Segmental Nervous Supply of Extremity Bones

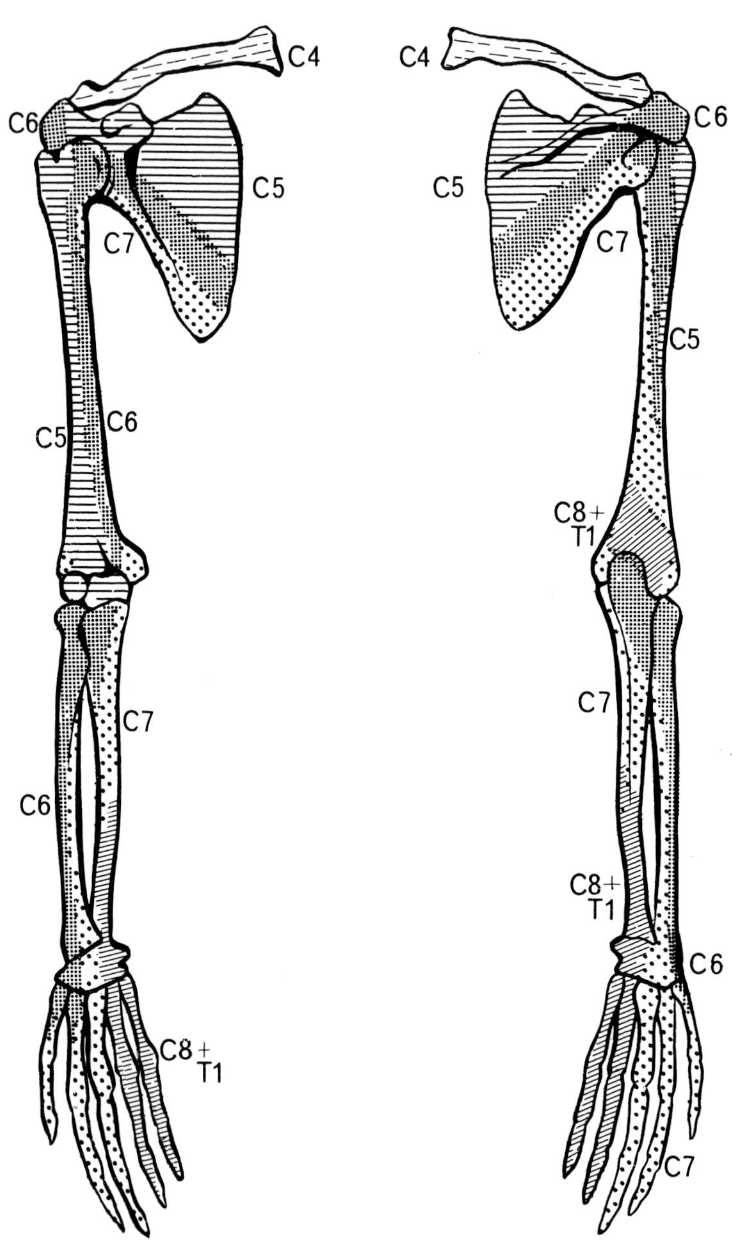

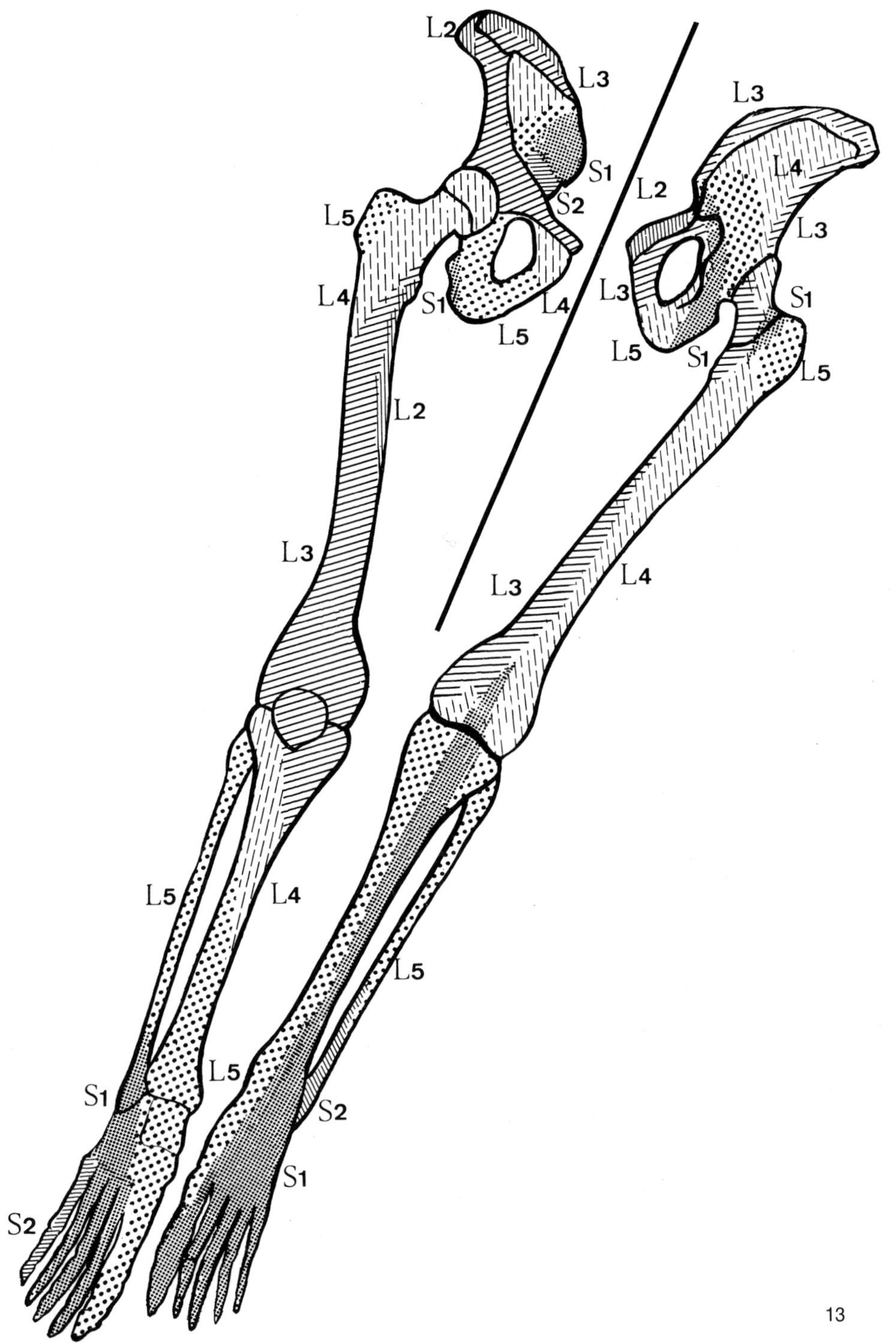

L2
L3
S1
S2
L5
L4
S1
L4
L5
L2
L3
L3
L4
L2
L3
L3
S1
L5
S1
L5
L3
L4
L5
L4
L5
L5
S1
S2
S1
S2

Peripheral Nerves Supplying Extremity Bones

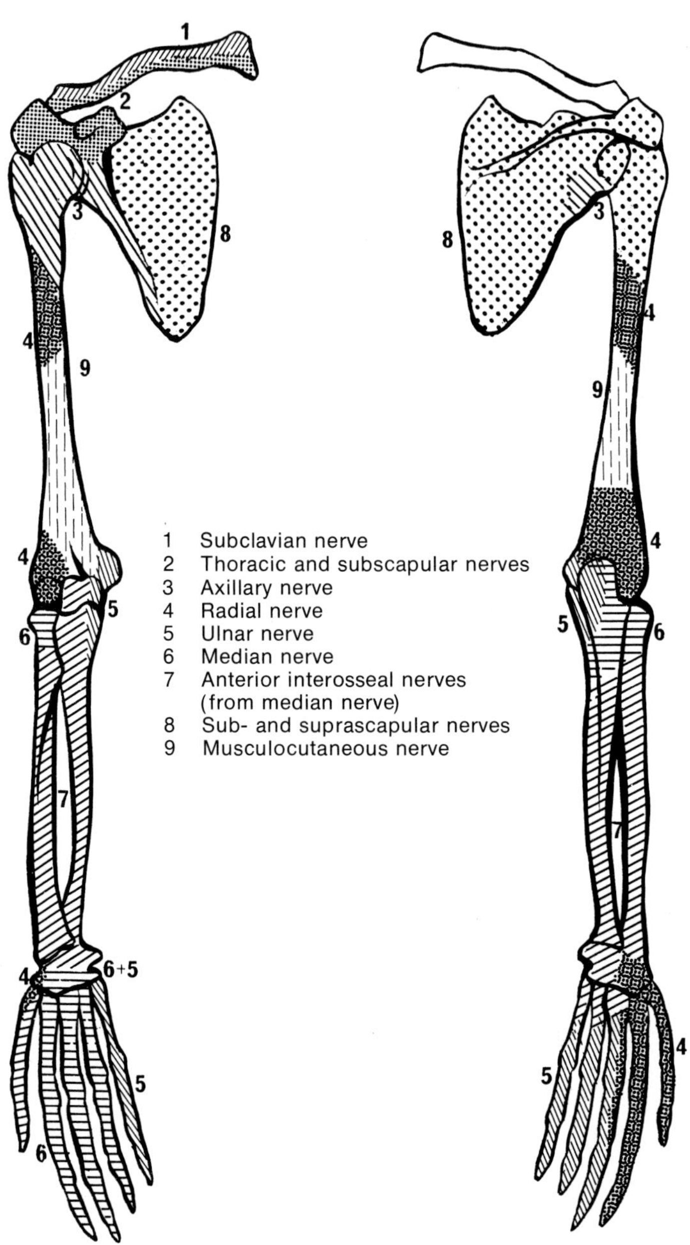

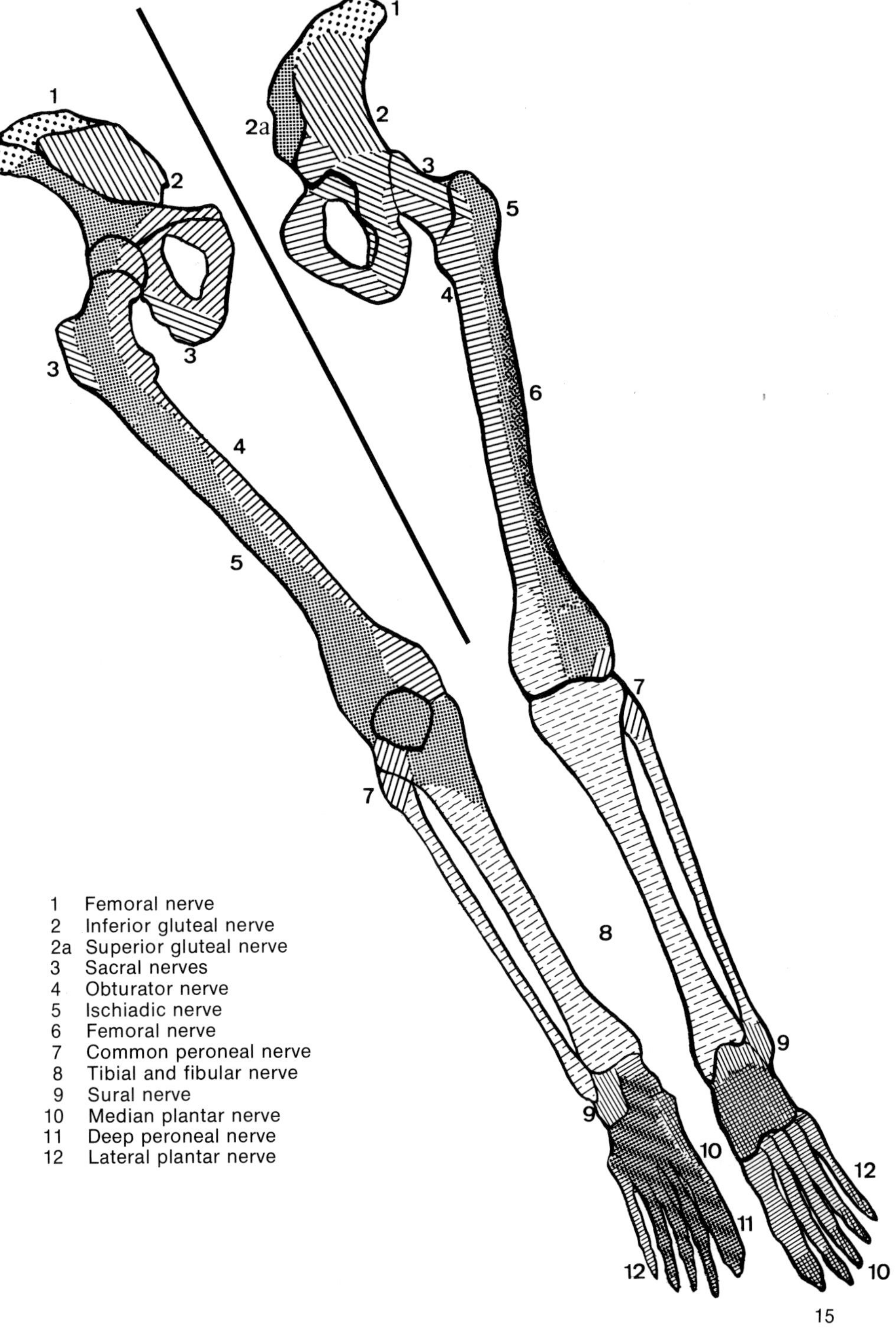

1 Femoral nerve
2 Inferior gluteal nerve
2a Superior gluteal nerve
3 Sacral nerves
4 Obturator nerve
5 Ischiadic nerve
6 Femoral nerve
7 Common peroneal nerve
8 Tibial and fibular nerve
9 Sural nerve
10 Median plantar nerve
11 Deep peroneal nerve
12 Lateral plantar nerve

Complications and Their Treatment

To keep to a minimum the number and kind of complications that may occur during use of any local anesthetic for blocks as well as any other procedure, it is advised that the following measures be adhered to.

Preparation of skin should be done as for an operation: surgical preparation. In more difficult and extensive blocks sterile gowns, gloves, and masks should be worn by the physician, as is customary for operations.

Paresthesias are always a sign that the respective nerve has been reached by the tip of the needle or that the tip of the needle is situated within the nerve. It is required that the needle be withdrawn a little because intraneural injections are not desired. The solution should be placed around the nerve.

Intravascular injections are to be avoided. It is absolutely necessary to aspirate before injecting. This has to be done in two planes, and for this the needle has to be turned around 180°. If the injection's planned for a very vascular area, aspiration in three planes (i. e., every 120°) is advised.

The value of **single maximum doses** seems doubtful to many, especially because the resorption of local anesthetics depends so much on the site of application, e. g. it varies for mucous membranes, bladder, trachea, and by injection for a nerve block. Nevertheless, it is advised that one attend to the single maximum doses for each drug, recalling at the same time that higher concentrations of a drug are resorbed much faster than lower concentrations (see page 5). When aspiration of the local anesthetic solution is done from a vial, the needle should never be left in the stopper.

Local Complications

Local edema, infection, abscesses, necroses, and gangrene are complications of an infectious nature caused by unsterile handling. Gangrene and ischemia are to be prevented if solutions containing no adrenaline or other vasoconstrictors are used. Contraindicated are any such admixtures in areas where endarteries exist, such as on fingers (Oberst's block). The simultaneous use of tourniquets with solutions containing adrenaline for obtaining bloodless fields is also contraindicated (fingers, toes, penis). As soon as there is a suggestion of damage by vasoconstrictors, one should not hesitate to apply vasodilators or block the respective part of the sympathetic chain immediately.

It should not be necessary to point out that only new, sharp needles should be used and that needles with hooks or other damage should not be used. One should not hesitate, where a needle is broken and a part remains in tissue, to remove this part, if necessary by surgery. Each needle has to be checked by the attending nurse before its use or in the case of longer needles before sterilization. It may be mentioned here that a double check on the contents of a syringe is advisable to prevent that other than local anesthetic substances (e. g. absolute alcohol) is injected. Injections of 96% percent alcohol usually are indicated only for cranial nerves.

General Complications

An overdose of a local anesthetic or allergic reactions to local anesthetics may lead to general complications which, according to their manifestations, are termed cardiovascular, neurologic, etc. If they appear immediately, they are called immediate reactions, but late reactions are just as frequent. Vascular reactions of the first type lead to cardiac failure, whereas the latter result in respiratory paralysis.

Overall, one may say that severe complications are extremely rare. Most toxic reactions occur when a local anesthetic is injected into a heavily vascularized area. Drugs and apparative requirements for therapeutic measures should be available at all times. In cases of severe, especially toxic incidences, an anesthesiologist should be consulted as soon as possible.

Individual symptoms are classified as to their causes as follows (after Moore):

Effect		on	Clinical picture
Effects on Central Nervous System	First stage: Stimulation of	Cortex Medulla	Agitation, disorientation, disturbances of speech, convulsions Vasomotor centrum: rise of blood pressure Respiratory center: faster rate of respiration, changes in rhythm of respiration Nausea and vomiting
	Second stage: Inhibition of	Cortex Medulla	Unconsciousness Vasomotor center: fall in blood pressure with fast pulse, or pulse not palpable (syncope) Respiratory center: arrhythmic respirations or apnea
Peripheral Effects	Organs	Heart Vessels	Bradycardia (= direct effect on myocardium; this effect is used therapeutically for arrhythmias) Vasodilation (direct effect on vessels)
	Allergic reactions	Skin Respiration Circulation	Urticaria Depression } clinically as Depression } anaphylactic shock

Varia:

1. Psychogenic reactions.
2. Reactions to other constituents, such as vasoconstrictors.

Active Measures in Case of Toxic Reactions

1. Watch for or establish free airway (suction, bronchial toilette).
2. O_2 (by mask or tube) and support respiration, if necessary.
3. Start infusion immediately at onset of reaction (if only to have intravenous channel available on demand).
4. Terminate convulsions
   (a) sometimes by O_2 only
   (b) i. v. succinylcholinchloride, 40 mg, or
   (c) thiopental, 50 mg, every 1 to 2 min until convulsions have terminated
   (d) with artificial respiration.
5. Reestablish normal blood pressure level, if necessary, by external cardiac massage.

Equipment required: O_2, suction, endotracheal tubes, airways, laryngo- and bronchoscopes, electrocardiograph, defibrillator; drugs: vasoconstrictors, succinylcholinchloride, short-acting barbiturates, corticosteroids, antihistaminics, KCl, and procainamid.

Untoward Incidences

Untoward incidences are possible with all applications of any local anesthetic, be it for surface anesthesia, infiltration anesthesia, field block, nerve block, spinal anesthesia, intravenous anesthesia, intravenous use of local anesthetic for overshooting vegetative reaction, as antiarrhythmic, entiepileptic, or as supplement to general anesthesia. Severe reactions of a toxic nature are practically always caused by faulty technique, wrong application, or overdosage. This means when absolute or relative overdose leads to too high a blood level of the respective anesthetic, neurologic, psychic, cardiovascular, or respiratory reactions may occur. The most severe incidences, such as coma, cardiac or respiratory arrest, cardiac failure, or convulsions, may be prevented by adhering closely to the suggestions given so far and with every block. It is absolutely essential to pay attention to single maximum doses and prevention of intravascular injections; and to be in constant readiness to undertake appropriate measures should first signs of beginning complications appear.

Dizzyness, sleepiness, or disturbed speech may indicate such an approaching comatose state. Weak pulse, perhaps irregular pulse, pale face, perspiration, and moist and cool hands may be interpreted as oncoming syncope and require appropriate measures. Breathlessness, short breath interrupted by some deep respirations, dyspnoe, short intervals of apnea, and the like are definite warnings of a possible respiratory arrest. Unrest, tremor, or facial twitchings may warn of oncoming generalized convulsions. To watch for signs like these will enable the practitioner to start appropriate preventive measures in time. Only prompt action will secure a successful outcome.

Allergic reactions have practically disappeared since procaine and other substances of the ester type have been replaced by drugs of the amide type. Itching, weals, edema (mainly of eyelids), drop of blood pressure, asthma, or very rarely an anaphylactic shock may be observed. Urticaria, joint pain, and all other known allergic manifestations may occur.

From a preventive point of view, the practice of raising a skin weal has its merits even if – for technical reasons – this might not be required: By waiting a while, hypersensitivity reactions may become evident and one does not have to rely on the patients statements. However, as in medicine in general, this again does not provide insurance against undue reactions.

Other Applications of Local Anesthetics

1. **Surface Anesthetics:**
   Surface anesthetics are special substances that penetrate skin and mucous membranes with ease; examples are cocaine for the eye, quinisocaine for skin and mucous membranes.
2. **Infiltration Anesthesia**
3. **Field Block:**
   Only weak concentrations of local anesthetics are used for these two techniques. They are suitable only for small procedures, mainly because relatively large amounts of anesthetics are necessary for complete analgesia. Be careful never to use more than single maximum doses (which is not necessary when blocking nerves)!
4. **Spinal Anesthesia:**
   Special high-percentile solutions, either heavier than CSF (then called "heavy") or lighter than CSF (then called "light") are used exclusively.
5. **Intrevenous Anesthesia:**
   Initiated by Bier (1908), this technique has recently been revived (Holmes, 1963; Bell, 1963; Adams, 1964; Marrifield, 1965; Eriksson, 1966). Is applied only to extremities. Injection is done into bloodless extremity after a tourniquet has been placed and a pressure of between 50 and 150 mm Hg over arterial systolic pressure maintained. Only 0.5 percent solutions of short-acting drugs and without adrenaline are to be used. For an arm, the dosage is 2 to 3 mg/kp of body weight, which

amounts to about 40 ml; for a leg, the dosage is 5 to 6 mg/kp of body weight, i. e., about 60 ml. Suffiσient muscular relaxation and anesthesia is achieved 10 to 15 min after injection. The tourniquet must stay in place a minimum of 15 min, otherwise increased side effects are observed. A maximum of 30 to 40 min of uninterrupted pressure is advised; longer placement leads to unpleasant sensations. The absolute upper limit of application time for tourniquet is 1 to 1.5 hr. Normal sensation returns 2 to 5 min after removal of the tourniquet.

6. **Antiarrhythmic:**
   Ventricular (not supraventricular) extrasystoles may be influenced successfully by intravenous lidocaine or mepivacaine. Initial dose is 20 to 50 mg, up to 100 mg, the latter only under direct ECG monitoring. Injection has to be done slowly (1 to 2 min) and may be followed by infusion, 1 to 2 mg/min, because a single injection acts only for 10 to 20 min. For infusions, ECG monitoring is also advisable. Signs of overdosage are prolongation of PQ interval of broadening of QRS complex. Only solutions without adrenaline are suitable. Oral application is under investigation, but because of uncertain resorption and short duration it is not advisable. As contraindications, severe liver damage and myasthenia gravis are known. Even though coronary infarction is a good indication for use of local anesthetics, a general application in case of every fresh infarction is not advised, even though it is being discussed. 4.5 mg/kg of body weight of lidocaine into the deltoid muscle deep i. m. results in a blood level of 2.8 mg, which is reported to be the lowest level necessary for prophylaxis of arrhythmias according to Schwartz et al. (XIIth International Congress of Diseases of Chest, London, July 7–12, 1974).
7. **Antiepileptic:**
   Local anesthetics cause epileptiform convulsions if an overdose is given. Nevertheless, 2 to 4 mg/kp of body weight (given i. v.) of lidocaine are used to cope with epileptic seizures in status epilepticus. This injection is equivalent to 10 mg/kg of pentobarbital (nembutal) in its antiepileptic effect. Only solutions without adrenaline are suitable. As an example, usually 2 to 3 mg/kp are injected within 30 to 45 sec. If no effect ensues, the patient is refractory. If the effect is sufficient, the injection should be followed by an infusion of 6 to 8 mg/kp/hr during 2 to 3 hr, with a maximum dose of 10 mg/kp/hr.
8. **General Applications:**
   In cases of overshooting vegetative reactions, Menière's disease, testing vestibular function, or for otosclerosis operations, i. v. therapy has been used. Dosage is like that given for antiepileptic use. Eichholtz has advocated 1 g of procaine in 500 ml of 0.9 percent NaCl (= 2 percent solution) to be infused slowly over about 2 hr in cases of serum sickness or similar allergic reactions and has reported dramatic results.

Relative Frequency of Some of the More Important Blocking Procedures

Blocking Procedure	Over all relative frequency	Relative frequency in benign : malignant diseases
Stellate block	3.5	6 : 1
Lumbar sympathetic block	3.5	2 : 1
Occipital (maj.) block	1.25	4 : 1
Deep cervical plexus	6.5	1 : 1
Intercostal block	1.5	3 : 2
Paravertebral thoracic somatic nerve block	15.5	1 : 1
Paravertebral lumbar somatic nerve block	6.5	2 : 1
Sacral nerve block	3	1 : 7
Epidural segmental block	1.5	none all
Obturator block	1.7	all none
Local infiltration (joints)	0.75	all none

Special Section

Guidelines to Presentation of Individual Blocks

Indications

This paragraph gives a listing of a wide range of useful indications for each block, even though not all authors agree on all of these. The reader may make his selection or try out all.

1. **Diagnostic:** For these indications use short (fast)-acting drugs. Plan procedure as a step toward correct diagnosis.
2. **Therapeutic:** For these indications use long-acting drugs. Depending on purpose, select concentration of drug: lowest concentration for sympathetic (vasomotor) block, highest concentration for complete sensory and motor block.
3. **Surgical:** If possible, use long-acting drugs. In some procedures, no surgical application is possible; this is clearly stated.

Technique

This paragraph describes the various steps of the procedure in sequence.

1. **Possibilities:** If more than one approach is possible, the most useful (not always the easiest) procedure is described. Occasionally, alternative procedures or approaches are presented, indicating advantages or disadvantages. Sometimes, alternative blocks (of other structures) are indicated.
2. **Positioning** of a patient always is of utmost importance. One should never underestimate it.
3. **Landmarks** give points of orientation essential for proper execution of individual block.
4. **Point of block** indicates at which site along the course of a nerve a block should be carried out.
5. **Procedure** gives step-by-step description from cleansing of skin and skin wealing (optional) to withdrawal of needle after injection is finished. Precautionary measures are mentioned at end of this paragraph.

Evaluation of Effect: Hints for how to make sure if block is working or not.

Complications: The more common and also some of the rarest complications that may occur at respective block are given.

Local Anesthetic: Quantities of solution to be used preferably for respective block are indicated specifically for fast-acting (see page 5) drugs; figures in brackets refer to long-acting drugs, such as bupivacaine.

Onset and Duration: For the same most diverging groups of drugs the figures are given approximately. Again, figures in brackets are for long-acting drugs.
(The more experienced will need less anesthetic and still obtain faster and longer effect, because good averages are given).

Stellate Ganglion Block

Indications

1. **Diagnostic:** Differentiating various vasospastic conditions of arm and head, cardiac disease, and some forms of asthma. In prognosticating effectiveness or cervico-thoracic sympathectomy. Evaluating some causes of so-called cervical vertebral syndrome (arm-shoulder syndrome).

2. **Therapeutic:**
   (a) To influence vasospastic states of arm, face, brain, and lung; arterial dysfunction (such as scalenus anticus syndrome, Volckmann's contracture, Raynaud's disease, Buerger-Winiwarter's disease, thromboses or embolisms of arm, lung, or brain); venous dysfunction (thrombophlebitic, postphlebitic edema); mixed forms (e. g., lymphedema of arm, such as may occur after amputation of female breast), cold trauma of arms, cervical migraine, Menière's disease.

   (b) In treatment of posttraumatic dystrophies of bone, posttraumatic osteoporosis, causalgia, phantom pain of arm, hyperhidrosis of upper half of body.

   (c) To assist in therapy of painful conditions where positive influence seems possible by severing of sympathetic chain, such as, e. g., slow-healing ulcers, herpes zoster, anginoid states, asthmatic states; to assist in healing of plastic surgical procedures on arm, neck, or face when circulation is insufficient; in cardiac decompensation, because depressed ST interval of ECG is elevated to normal by stellate block; subacromial bursitis, epicondylitis; in cases of pulmonary edema bilateral block should be performed or tried; as adjunct in the therapy of cerebral edema.

3. **Surgical:** none.

Technique

1. **Possibilities:** There are more than 34 methods from anterior, antero-lateral, lateral, supero-lateral, and posterior possible. The most simple, safe, and problem-free is the approach from the anterior. Only patients who do not tolerate hyperextension of the cervical spine should be approached anterolaterally.

2. **Position of Patient:** reclined, with pillow under shoulders and cervical spine hyperextended, as shown in figure on page 26.

3. **Landmarks:** Pomum adami, anterior border of sternocleidomastoid muscle, and jugular notch. In normally built people the method of the figure on page 26 gives the point of piercing of skin. In people with stout or short necks this point must be modified, but not too far laterally.

4. **Point of Block:** Stellate ganglion, which is usually situated anterior to the transverse process of the seventh cervical vertebra or anterior to the head of the first rib.

5. **Procedure:** Advise the patient not to speak or swallow during the procedure and not to change his position. After cleansing and wealing (usually not necessary) of skin, a 5-cm needle always on a filled 5 (or 10)-ml syringe and filled with solution is advanced in an exact vertical direction until bone contact is made. This always occurs in less than 3.5 cm of depth. If at this depth no bone is met, withdraw the needle to beneath the skin and advance it in a slightly different (cranial) direction. Sometimes, if no bone is met, paresthesias of brachial plexus are felt. In this case withdraw the needle and change position as well. If bone is met, withdraw the needle 0.5 or 1 mm, aspirate, and slowly inject 5 mm of local anesthetic. This will flood not only the stellate ganglion but sometimes also the middle and superior cervical ganglia and the upper two or three thoracic ganglia of the sympathetic chain of the same side.

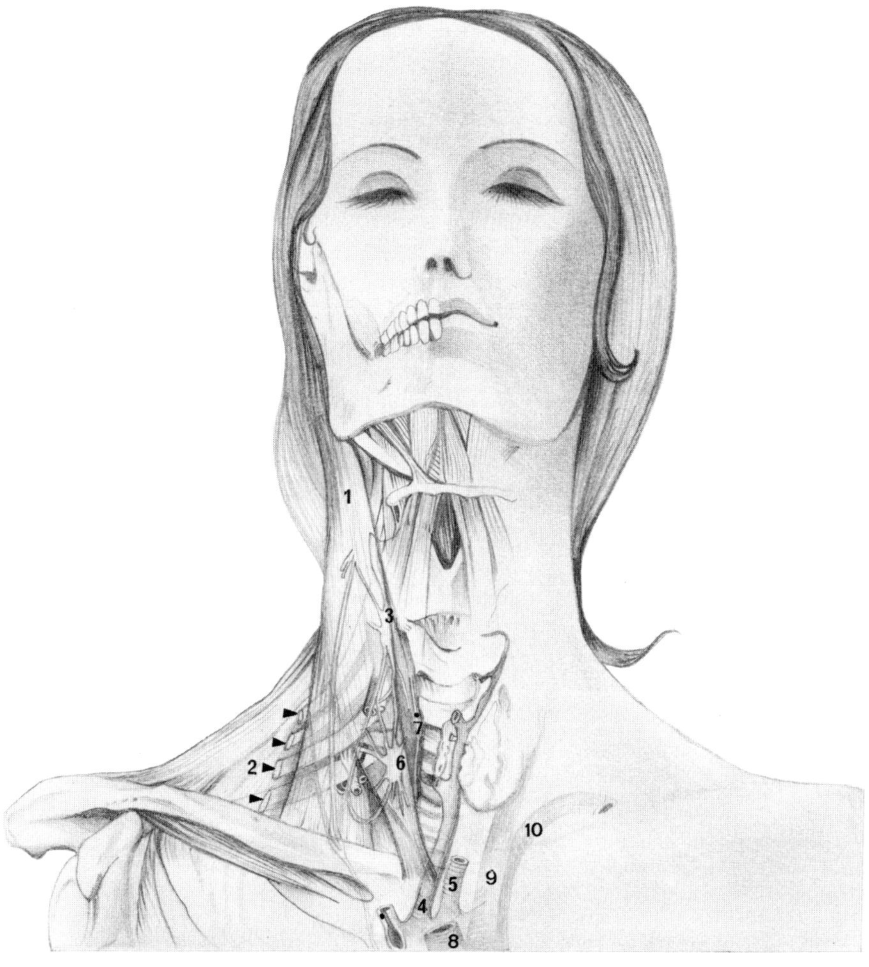

1 Sternocleidomastoid muscle
2 Brachial plexus
3 Middle cervical ganglion
4,5 Thyroid veins
6 Stellate ganglion
7 Recurrent nerve
8 Brachiocephalic trunc
9 Left common carotid artery
10 Subclavian artery

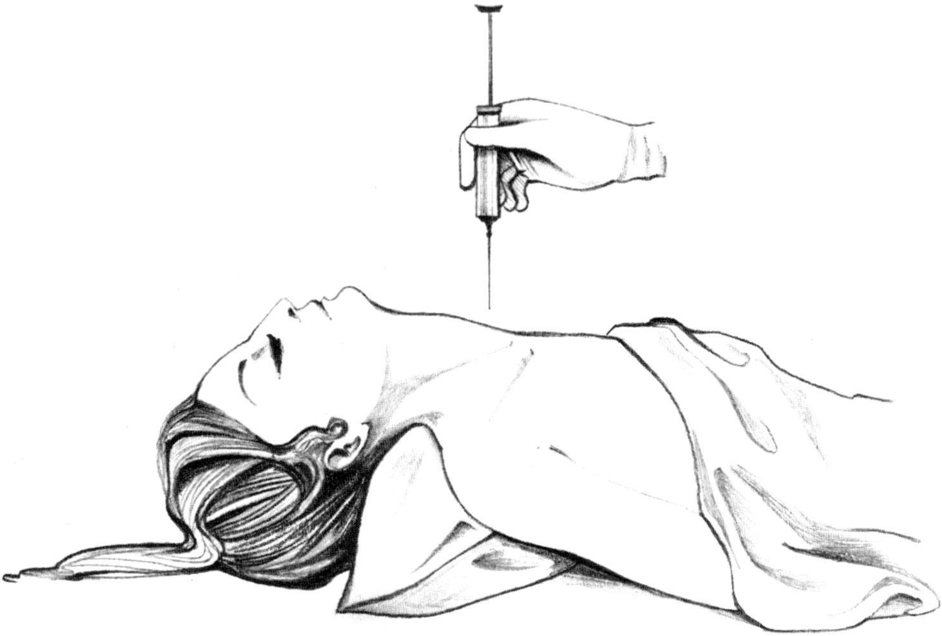

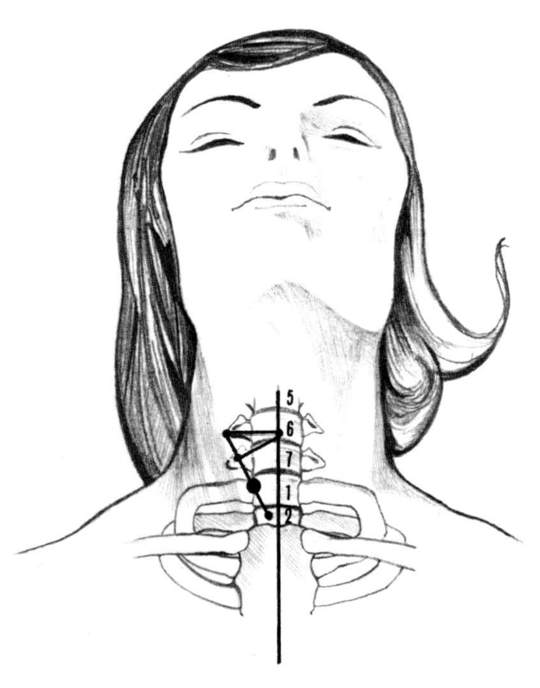
5
6
7
1
2

Evaluation of Effect: Evaluation of effect is possible by observing the patient immediately after or even during injection for the following signs: miosis, ptosis, enophthalmus (= Horner's syndrome), and a little later conjunctival injection, increase of tear secretion, increase in skin temperature of face, arm, and hand, with slight reddening and anhidrosis (dry skin) of these areas and (sometimes) congestion of nose.

Complications: Complications are seen very rarely. Unimportant, even though somewhat irritating to the patient, are concomitant block (and paresis) of recurrent nerve (coarse voice, 5 to 8 percent), of parts of the brachial plexus (5 percent) and phrenic nerve; these all clear within hours. Puncture of the thyroid gland is of no importance. Puncture of the carotid artery (which may be easily recognized by pulsations of the needle) is of no consequence; slight pressure may be applied locally for a short while. Injections into the vertebral artery (which are to be prevented by aspiration) will lead to incoordination of ocular movements (as a first sign) immediately followed by subjective ear noises and vertigo and – if injection is not stopped – by convulsions, arrest of respiration, and irregularities of cardiac action. Therefore, observing the eyes will allow one to observe the effect of the block by decreasing size of pupils on the side of injection and also showing the first signs of lack of coordination of ocular movements as a first sign of intraarterial (vertebral) injection. Sometimes a swallowing movement may bring a correctly placed needle tip to pierce the artery during injection, and therefore observing the eyes is mandatory. The only serious inadvertant side effect is puncture of the pleura with consective pneumothorax. It may occur very rarely but even to the experienced. Immediate measures should then be taken. The use of a needle filled with solution should prevent this complication.

Local Anesthetic: A solution of 5 ml of short-acting drug should be used; adrenaline should never be used. Some practitioners mix 5 ml of anesthetic with 5 ml of periston N. Long-acting (more toxic because of possible intraarterial injection) substances such as bupivacaine should never be used.

Onset and Duration: During injection, or several minutes after the end of injection at the latest, Horner's syndrome has to appear. The other signs such as skin reddening and increase in skin temperature may appear up to 30 min later, and should last 2 to 6 hr. They may last up to a day or longer. Most therapeutic indications require one to perform a series of blocks, usually five on one side and one on the opposite side; sometimes as much as 12 to 18 blocks may be necessary. Usually, the effect of a series of five blocks done every or every other day will last about a year. As an objective observation, the oscillatory index of the arm or rheogram of the arm or rheoencephalogram may be used; amplitudes of all these will increase following the block.

Survey of Some of the Better-Known Methods:

Approach	Anterior	Anterolateral	Lateral	Superolateral	Posterior
Author	Findley Herget	Leriche (1934)	Goinard (1934)	Arnulf	Mandl (1925)
Piercing of skin	3 cm cephalad of sterno-clavicular joint 1.5 cm lateral of trachea	2 cm cephalad of midpoint of clavicle, 45° tilted to sagittal plane	Anterior to border of trapezius muscle	Chassigny's tubercle (tip of transverse process of sixth cervical vertebra)	4 cm lateral of spin. process of sixth cervical vertebra, 25° tilt to sagittal and 15° to transverse
Length of needle	5 cm	8 cm	8 cm	5 cm	8–10 cm
Smallest amount	5 ml	5 ml	5 ml	5 ml	5 ml

Deep Cervical Plexus Block

Indications

1. **Diagnostic:** Differentiating various neuralgias of head, neck (C_2, $C_{3,4}$) and shoulder (C_5) regions.
2. **Therapeutic:** Relief of occipital headache and certain neck-shoulder pain.
3. **Surgical:** None.

Technique

1. **Possibilities:** Preferably by the lateral approach. Posterior approach is much more difficult to perform.
2. **Position:** Reclining, without pillow, head turned to contralateral side as far as possible.
3. **Landmarks:** Skin marks over mastoid process and anterior tubercle of transverse process of sixth cervical vertebra (= Chassaignac's tubercle, carotid tubercle), which is the most prominent transverse process of the cervical spine. These marks are connected by a line and some 0.7 to 1 cm posterior to this line, skin weals are raised and needles enter skin: for C-2 about 1.5 cm caudal of mastoid process and for each consecutive process 1 to 1.5 cm caudal thereof. This block should be carried out only if transverse process in respective segment may be identified and palpated. Otherwise – as may happen in people with short necks – do not try to perform block.
4. **Point of Block:** Respective cervical nerve, as it leaves notch of transverse process. This site lies 1.5 to 3 cm beneath the skin, the uppermost nerve being the deepest.
5. **Procedure:** After positioning the patient exactly, palpating transverse process and cleansing and skin wealing is done. A very thin needle, 3 to 5 cm in length, is advanced in a somewhat caudal direction to prevent dural puncture. In case of paresthesias, the needle is arrested immediately. Aspiration is done with a dry (empty) syringe (CSF!). Injection of 3 to 5 ml of local anesthetic per segment follows.

Evaluation of Effect: In most instances paresthesias are felt in occipitomastoideal (C-2), lateral nuchal region (C-3), or over clavicle (C-4). Testing of hypalgesia is done with needle point as usual.

Complications: If too much anesthetic solution is used (8 ml or more per segment), diffusion of solution to (and blocking of) vagus, hypoglossal, and accessory nerves (for C-2) leading to temporary increase in pulse frequency, aphonia, and weakness in shoulder lifting ensues. Phrenic nerve is involved from C-3, 4, and 5 and causes temporary paresis of the diaphragm on the same side. When aspirating clear fluid, which happens only when the needle is pointing cranially, the dural sack has been punctured and the needle has to be withdrawn and the block terminated as a trial only.

Local Anesthetic: 3 ml (higher concentration, longer-acting drug) to 5 ml (short-acting drug) per segment. Preferably without adrenaline.

Onset and Duration: 2 to 5 (to 10) min to full effect; 1.5 to 3 hr duration with short-acting drug. May be repeated with 96 percent alcohol, but this usually is not necessary when using a long-acting drug, which then carries the effect over 12 to 16 hr.

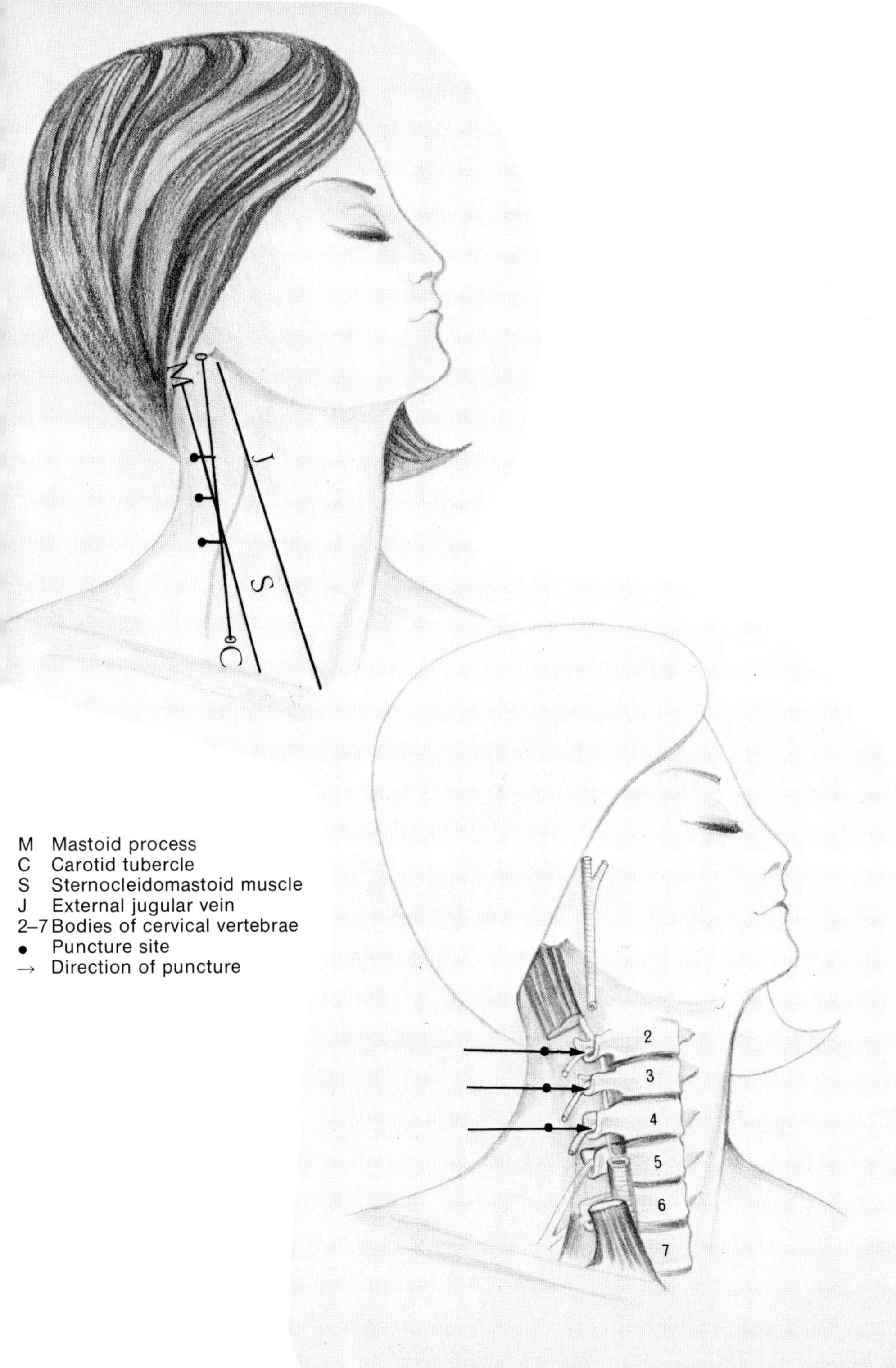

M
J
S
C
2
3
4
5
6
7
M Mastoid process
C Carotid tubercle
S Sternocleidomastoid muscle
J External jugular vein
2–7 Bodies of cervical vertebrae
● Puncture site
→ Direction of puncture

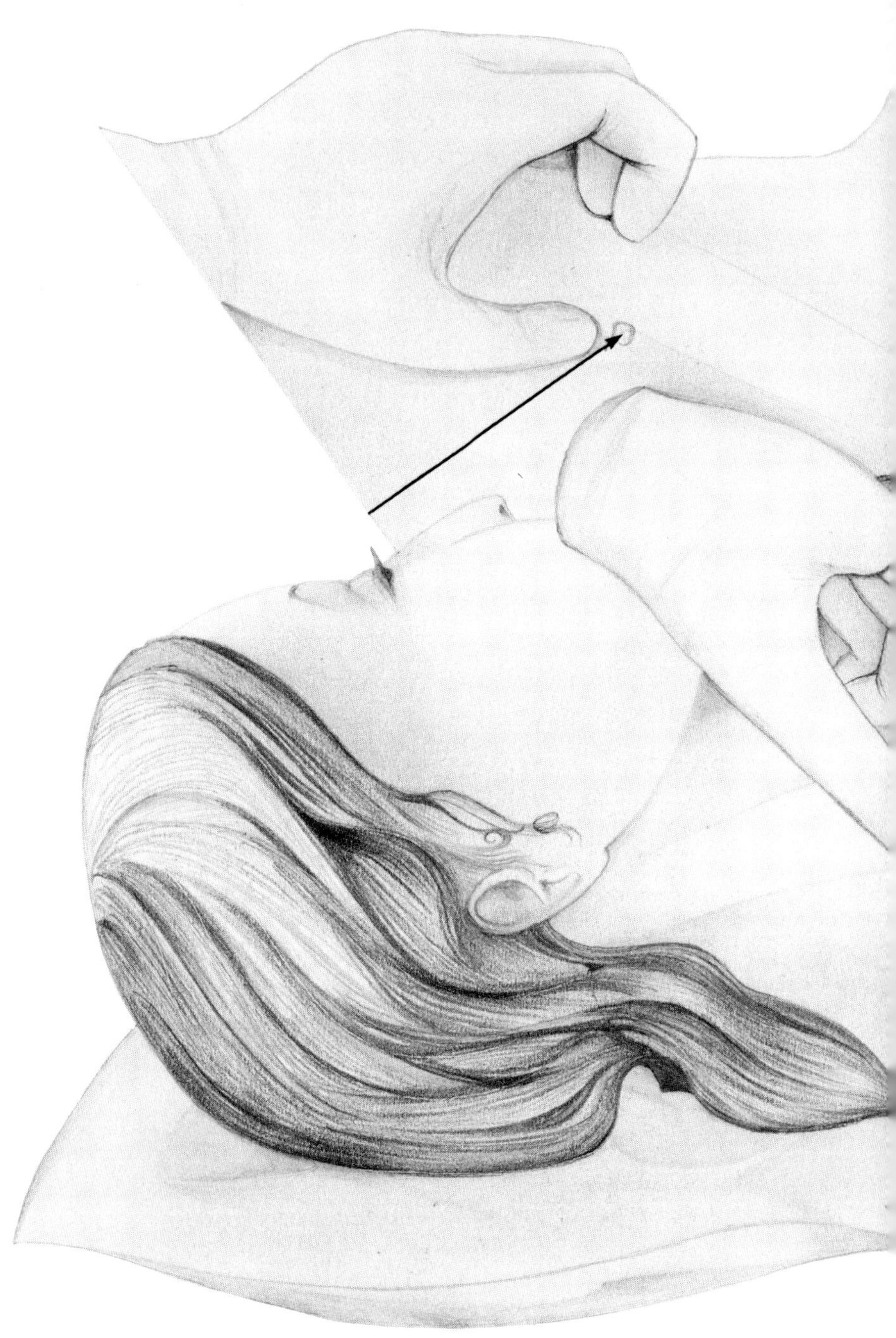

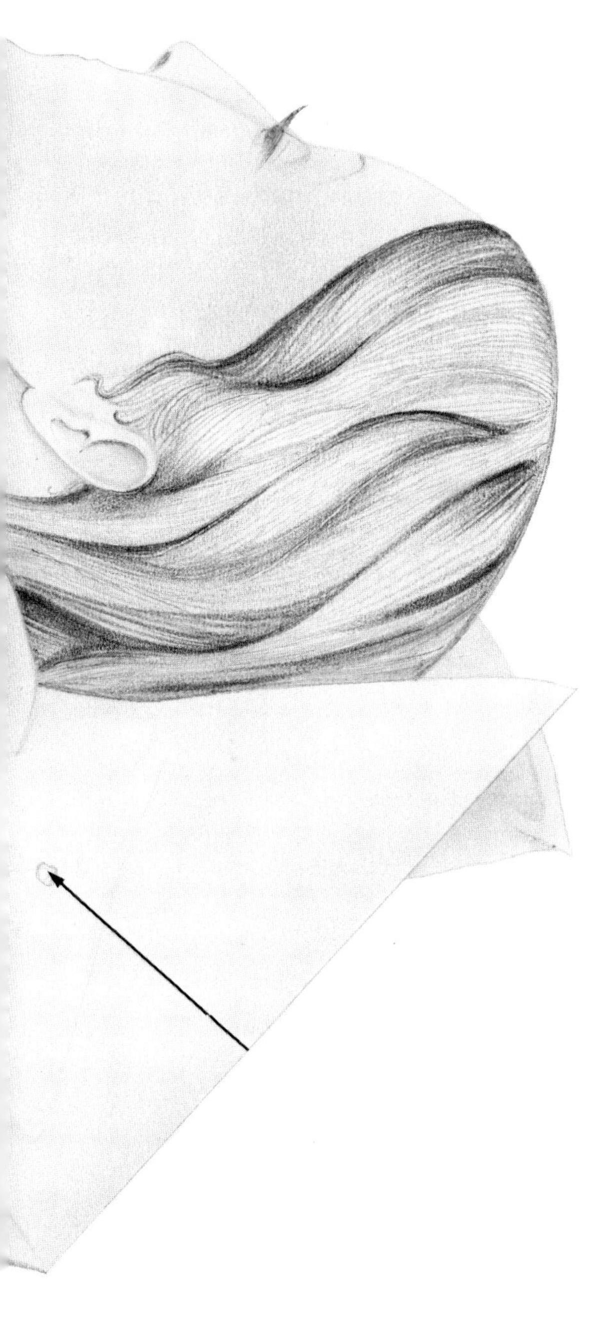

Phrenic Nerve Block

Indications

1. **Diagnostic:** To prognosticate the effect of severing or crushing the phrenic nerve.
2. **Therapeutic:** For alleviation of persistent singultus (hiccups).
3. **Surgical:** Occasionally to arrest motions of the diaphragm intraoperatively.

Technique

1. **Approach:** Percutaneous or at open thorax (see Indications, 3).
2. **Position:** Supine position, reclined, without a pillow, head turned to contralateral side.
3. **Landmarks:** Lateral part of clavicular head of sternocleidomastoid muscle, as well as scalenus anterior muscle 2 to 2.5 cm from clavicle (better visible if patient raises head a little).
4. **Point of Block:** Phrenic nerve, just under sternocleidomastoid.
5. **Procedure:** A skin weal is raised on the lateral border of the sternocleidomastoid muscle 2 cm cranial to clavicle after cleansing of skin. Thumb and index finger of left hand pull muscle from lodge of carotid (if operator is right-handed; there is a slight difference in position of hand depending on side of patient). Then a short (3.5–cm) needle on a 10 ml syringe is inserted through the skin weal and advanced behind the sternocleidomastoid muscle for a distance of 2 or 2.5 cm in a transveral plane in such a way that it comes to lay between the named and the scalenus anticus muscle. The finger on the medial side of the sternocleidomastoid may control the position of the needle. After careful aspiration up to 10 ml are slowly injected while gradually withdrawing the needle. **Note:** an alternative procedure is a block of the deep cervical plexus at C(3), 4 (and 5). Never perform a bilateral block of the phrenic nerve.

Evaluation: The only visible effect is arrest of the motion of the diaphragm on the same side. To be observed on deep respiration or fluoroscopy.

Complications: None. An occasional diffusion of the drug to the stellate ganglion may lead to Horner's syndrome; to recurrent nerve leads to coarse voice for a limited time. Both clear after some hours. If steps of procedure are observed, no intravascular injection or pneumothorax may be caused.

Local Anesthetic: 10 ml of a short-acting anesthetic in 1 or 2 percent solution or 5 to 8 ml of a longer-acting drug. The use of adrenaline is not advised in this block.

Onset and Duration: 5 (to 15 in case of long-acting drug) min after blocking, the effect should be fully present and last for about 1.5 to 3 (4 to 8) hr.

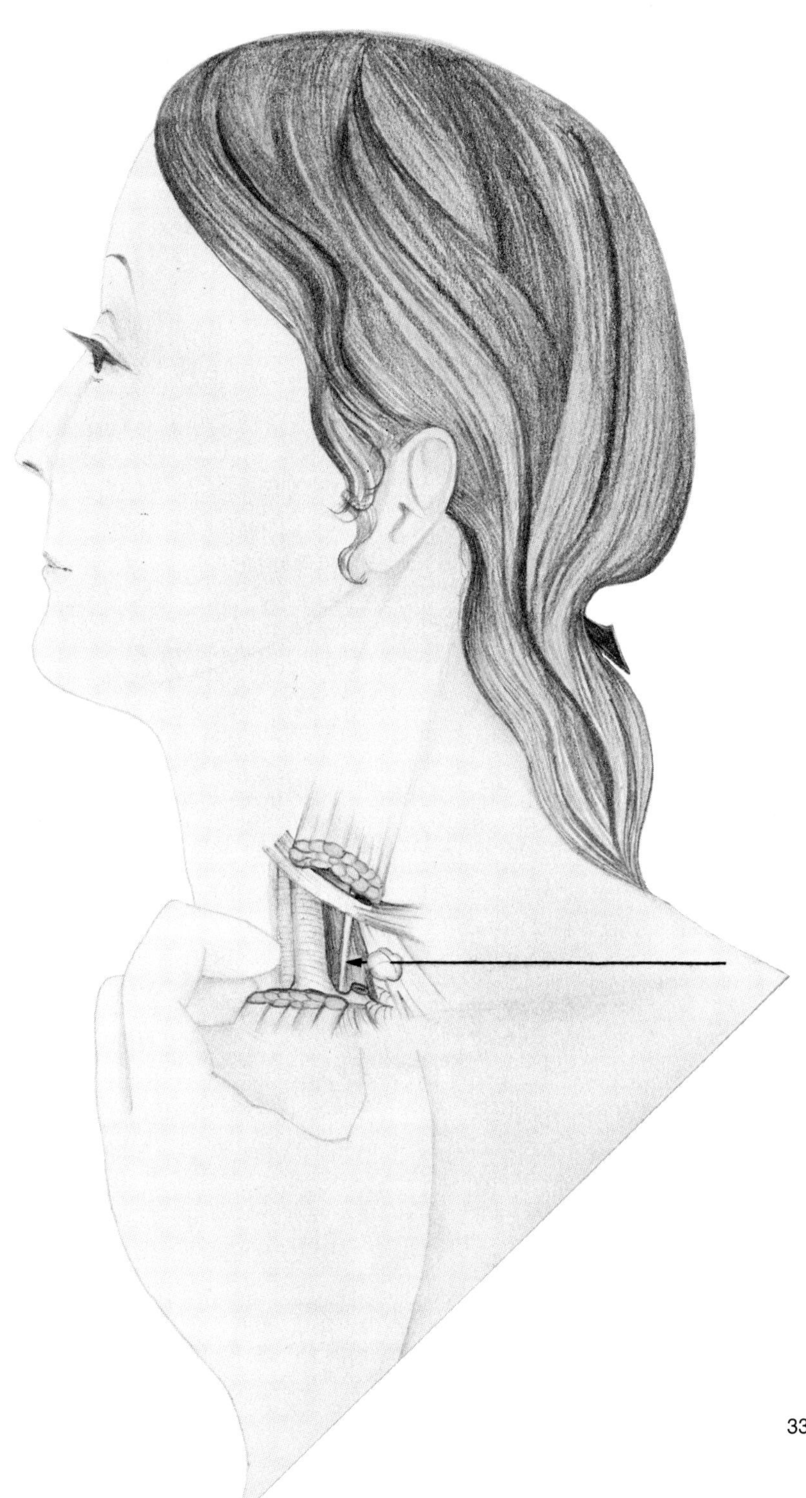

Brachial Plexus Block

Indications

1. **Diagnostic:** Differentiating organic from functional and central from peripheral painful states in the arm.

2. **Therapeutic:** Pain in distal third of upper arm and lower arm and hand; neuralgias, causalgia, pain from malignancy where metastatic infiltration of parts of plexus exists (then block may be carried out using 96 percent alcohol).

3. **Surgical:** For operations on lower arm and hand only. Reduction of dislocated shoulder only when using supraclavicular approach.

Technique

1. **Possibilities:** Supraclavicular, lateral paravertebral, posterior paravertebral, infraclavicular, and axillary approach. The last method does not give analgesia of the shoulder joint, but no danger of pneumothorax exists. The last but one method is most difficult to execute. Most often used are supraclavicular and axillary approaches.

2. **Position of Patient:** Reclining position, small pillow under upper thoracic spine to effectuate drop of shoulders. Turning of head to contralateral side and pulling homolateral arm caudal to achieve somewhat caudal position of same shoulder.

3. **Landmarks:** Midpoint of clavicle. Asking patient to raise head a little will mark the position of the posterior border of the anterior scalenus muscle. Subclavian artery and superficial jugular vein.

4. **Point of Block:** Brachial plexus in its course over first rib (approach A) or on humerus (approach B).

5. **Procedure:** (A) Supraclavicular approach. After marking and wealing skin 1 cm cephalad of clavicle, a 5 cm needle (0.8 mm caliber with short bevel) attached to a 10 ml syringe, both filled with solutions, is inserted through the weal in a somewhat medio-dorsal direction. It should point to the spinous process of the third thoracic vertebra. If paresthesias are provoked, the needle should be arrested immediately. This should be the case 1.5 to 2 cm below the skin. In no case should the needle be advanced more than 3 cm. Then inject 10 ml of solution slowly. Proceed to contact with first rib and inject another 10 ml while withdrawing needle to 1 cm beneath skin. If result is not satisfactory, another 7 to 10 ml may be injected behind the subclavian artery, advancing the needle somewhat more medio-posteriorly.

   Procedure: (B) Axillary approach. Reclining position with arm abducted 90° and elbow flexed 90°; arm is held in this position and patient is passive. Palpation of insertion of deltoid muscle on humerus. This marks the most peripheral plane of the block; more peripheral injections do not include the radial nerve distally. The neurovascular lodge is held in place. With the index and middle fingers of the left hand. After cleansing and wealing skin in the medial bicipital fold proximal to the mentioned plane, a 3.5 cm needle is advanced just anterior to the brachial artery. Injection of 10 ml of solution after aspiration. Then withdrawal of needle to place it posterior to artery and injection of another 10 ml (maximally). After up to 30 min, motor paresis of fingers and full analgesia should ensue. Duration over 3 hr.

Evaluation of Effect: Motor paresis of arm and finger muscles should appear. This is always the case if paresthesias have been provoked. However, one part of the plexus may be blocked and another not; then the block should be repeated, paying attention to the single maximum dose of the anesthetic used.

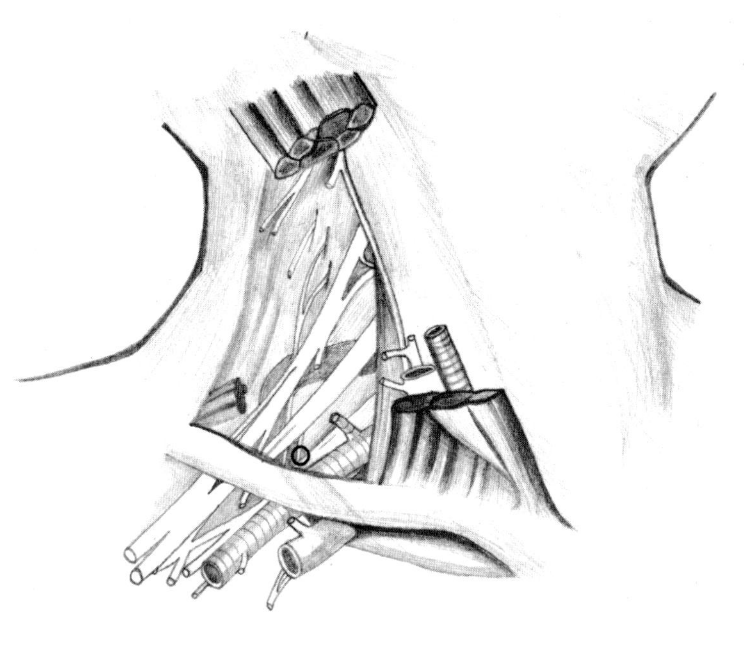

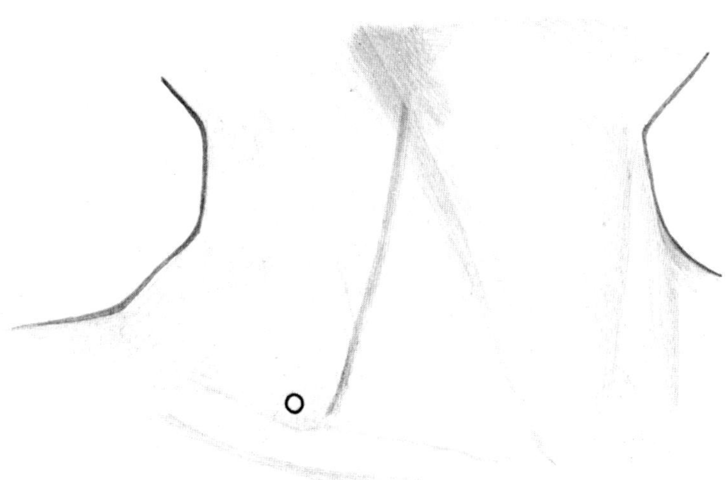

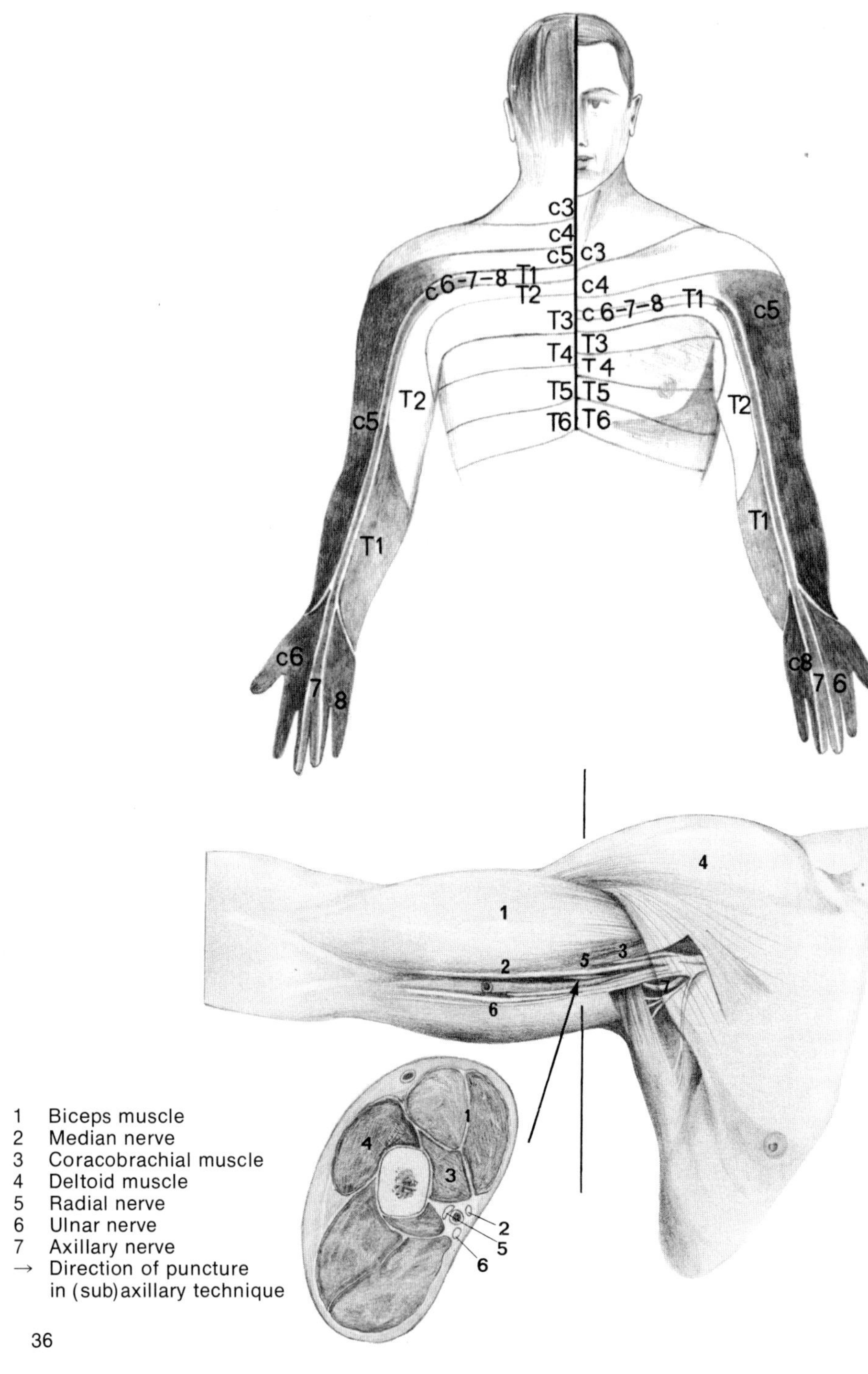

1 Biceps muscle
2 Median nerve
3 Coracobrachial muscle
4 Deltoid muscle
5 Radial nerve
6 Ulnar nerve
7 Axillary nerve
→ Direction of puncture in (sub)axillary technique

Complications: Pneumothorax [only with procedure (A)] in maximally 0.6 percent of cases, to be treated conservatively. Punctures of vessels are of no consequence, if properly handled; spreading of blocking solution to phrenic nerve (on unilateral block) or to stellate ganglion (*vide:* Horner!) clear after some hours. There is one contraindication for approach (A): This block should not be performed in a patient with pneumonectomy or lobectomy on normal (not-operated) side.

Local Anesthetic: 20 to 30 ml 1 percent lidocaine or 10 (15) ml of carbocaine (0.5 to 0.25 percent) with or without adrenaline may be used.

Onset and Duration: 5 to 10 to 20 min to full effect when using lidocaine and up to 30 min when using bupivacaine. Lasts for 2 to 4 hr with lidocaine and 5 to 16 hr with bupivacaine.

Ulnar Nerve Block

Indications

1. **Diagnostic:** In locating and differentiating painful states of upper extremity.
2. **Therapeutic:** See radial nerve block.
3. **Surgical:** Only for procedures on little finger and fifth metacarpal.

Technique

1. **Possibilities:** May be executed on elbow or wrist.
2. **Position:** Reclining position; for block at elbow: upper arm vertical to bed, in inward rotation and elbow flexed; at wrist: supinated hand.
3. **Landmarks:**

   At elbow
   Ulnar sulcus = groove between medial epicondyle and olecranon. Pressing here will cause paresthesias in little finger.

   At wrist
   Circular line around wrist at level of styloid process of ulna. Tendon of flexor carpi ulnaris muscle is seen or palpated when patient is closing fist firmly. At its radial side needle has to pierce skin. Lateral of it lies ulnar artery.

4. **Point of Block:** Ulnar nerve in ulnar sulcus or between ulnar artery and tendon of flexor carpi ulnaris muscle.
5. **Procedure**
   (a) **At Elbow:** After cleansing and wealing of skin at designated point, a 3 cm needle is advanced on a 5 ml syringe until paresthesias are elicited. This usually is the case at about 0.5 or 1.5 cm depth. If not, never advance needle more than 2.5 cm. At indication of paresthesias arrest needle and slowly inject 5 ml of solution, then withdraw needle. Block at elbow is much more effective than at wrist, and not only simpler, because 5 cm distal to site of block, the nerve divides up into a volar and dorsal branch; at wrist, only the volar branch is reached.
   (b) **At Wrist:** After cleansing and wealing of skin, a 3 cm needle is advanced perpendicular to skin surface, to a maximum depth of 2 cm. If paresthesias are elicited, needle is arrested, aspirated, and 5 ml are injected slowly. If no paresthesias are obtained, withdraw needle to just beneath skin and proceed in slightly different direction. In this block, the needle is affixed to a 10 ml syringe, because it is advisable to infiltrate intradermally and subcutaneously the dorsal half of the circumference of the wrist to reach the dorsal branch as well.

Evaluation: Only fifth finger becomes analgesic; test with needle tip.

Complications: None; if aspiration is not done, there may be intravascular injection at wrist, which is preventable.

Local Anesthetic: 5 ml of any anesthetic suffices; use 10 ml at wrist, if skin infiltration dorsally is done. Preferably do not use adrenaline.

Onset and Duration: After 2 min, short-acting drugs last about 1.5 to 3 hr. Long-acting drugs take 10 to 15 min to onset and last 6 to 12 hr.

Remark

On lower arm or hand, only a wound, procedure, or painful state on little finger may be made painless by a single block. For all other areas two or even three blocks become necessary, because there is large variation in supply and great overlapping innervation. In blocking single nerves, additional skin infiltration of large areas is occasionally necessary. Then it may become difficult to stay under the amount limited by the maximum single dose of drug. It then seems opportune to use a blocking procedure of a more proximal type like brachial plexus block. This is also advocated for operations where a turniquet is required for a bloodless field: If blocking peripheral to a turniquet, the pressure soon becomes unbearable.

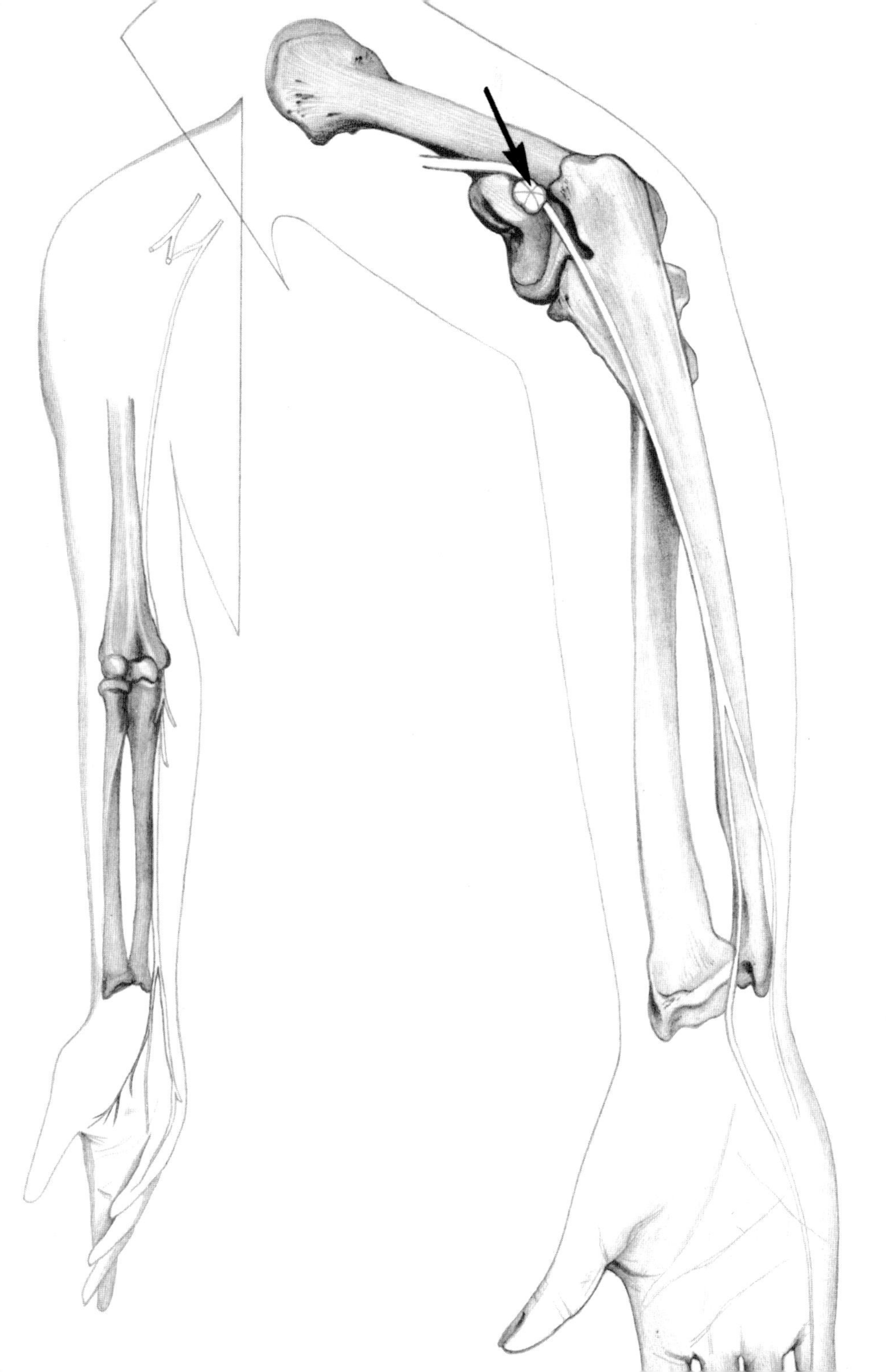

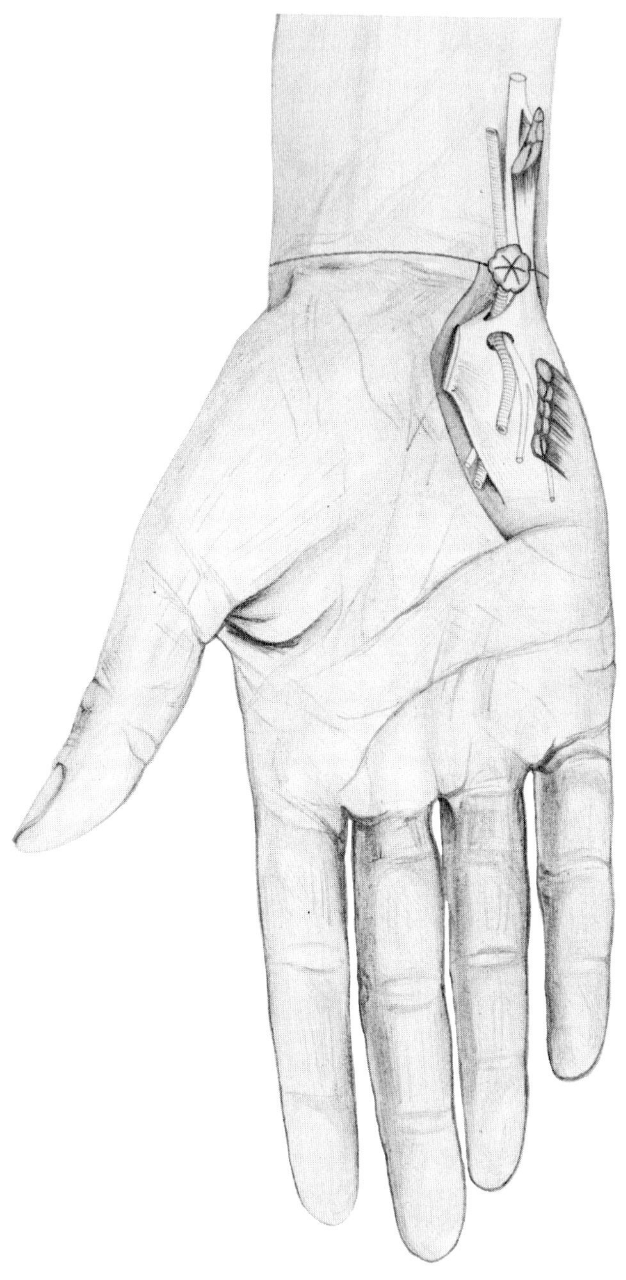

Median Nerve Block

Indications

1. **Diagnostic:** in evaluating painful states of forearm and hand.
2. **Therapeutic:** In treating pain and vasospastic states in the innervation area of the median nerve peripheral to the blocking site.
3. **Surgical:** For small procedures in the area innervated by median nerve.

Technique

1. **Possibilities:** At elbow or wrist.
2. **Position:**

At elbow

Reclining, arm abducted, elbow flexed, hand supinated.

At wrist

Reclining, arm abducted; for orientation: elbow flexed, fist closed; for blocking: elbow extended, hand supinated.

3. **Landmarks:**

At elbow

Just medial to where line connecting both condyles crosses brachial artery skin is marked.

At wrist

A volar circle around wrist is made at level of the styloid process of ulna. With fist closed firmly, tendon of palmaris longus (or flex. digig. subl.) muscle is visualized. Radial of this the skin is marked on the circle.

4. **Point of Block:**

Median nerve beneath skin mark (see sketch).

Median nerve beneath skin mark at site between tendons of palmaris longus and flexor carpi radialis muscles (see sketch).

5. **Procedure:** After cleansing and wealing skin 2 cm distal to skin mark, medial to brachial artery, a 5 cm needle on a filled 5 ml syringe is advanced; the needle is tilted 30° to the skin, pierced through lacertus fibrosus at midpoint to skin mark and advanced to level of skin mark; arrest needle with paresthesias. In case these are not voiced, withdraw needle to lacertus and reinsert with smaller tilt to level of skin mark. After aspiration inject 5 ml of solution slowly and withdraw needle.

At site of skin mark cleanse and weal skin. Insert a 2 or 3 cm needle perpendicular to the skin until paresthesias are initiated. Arrest needle, inject 5 ml of local anesthetic, and withdraw needle. If no paresthesias are felt, advance needle in a fan-like fashion several times after withdrawing to skin level, because the median nerve may be found behind the tendon of the flexor carpi radialis muscle.

Evaluation: Pin pricking in area of median nerve peripheral of block.

Complications: None.

Local Anesthetic: 5 ml of any solution.

Onset and Duration: After 2 to 5 (to 10) min, effect lasts about 1.5 to 3 (4 to 8) hr.

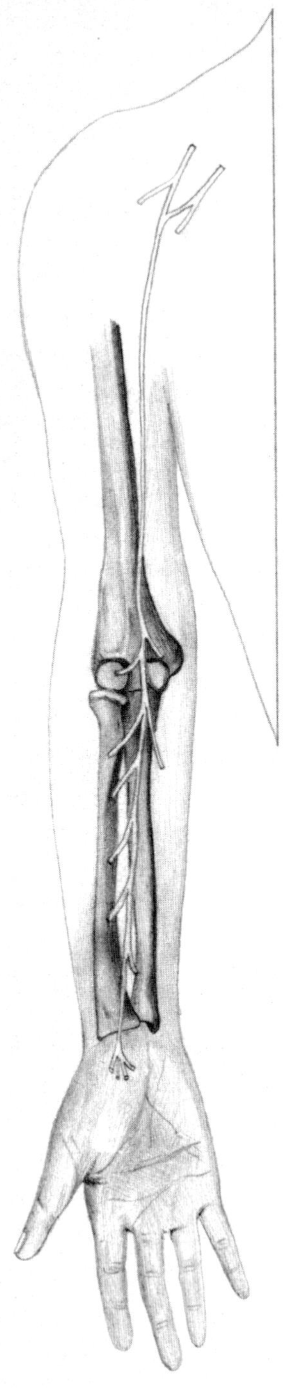
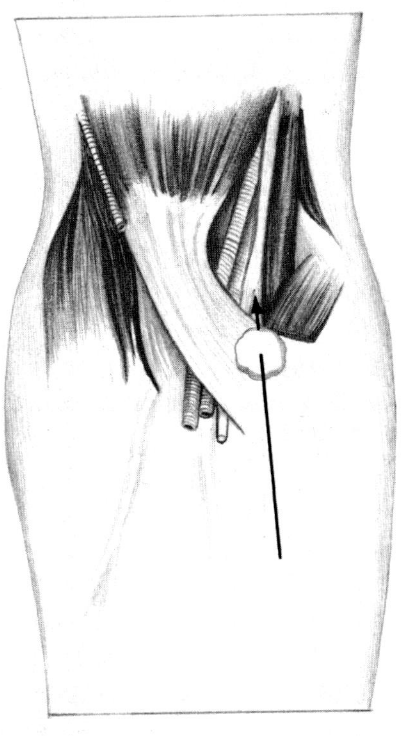

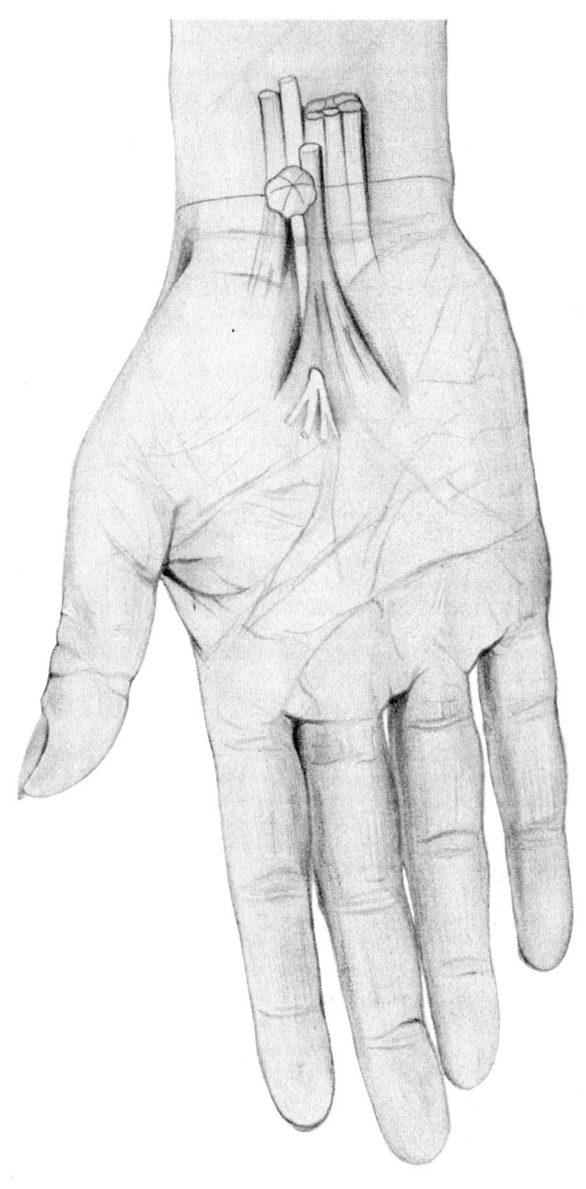

Radial Nerve Block

Indications

1. **Diagnostic:** In localizing and diagnosing painful states of upper extremity.
2. **Therapeutic:** Rarely, because all pain or vasospastic disorders exceed the innervation area of radial nerve. Therefore, the use of brachial plexus or stellate ganglion blocks is advised instead.
3. **Surgical:** None, except in small procedures in the area of the radial nerve innervation peripheral to block.

Technique

1. **Possibilities:** At elbow or wrist.
2. **Position:** In both cases reclined, arm partially abducted, forearm extended at elbow; when blocking at wrist, hand partially supinated.
3. **Landmarks:**

At elbow	At wrist
Skin is marked 6 to 7.5 cm proximal to lateral concyle for skin weal.	Circular line around wrist, at level of styloid process of ulna is drawn. Lateral (= radial) of radial artery skin is marked for weal.

4. **Point of Block:** Radial nerve beneath skin mark.
5. **Procedure:**
   (a) **At Elbow:** After cleansing and wealing of skin, a 5 cm short bevelled needle on a 5 (or 10)–ml syringe is advanced perpendicular to the skin at the site of the skin mark. Should paresthesias be felt, arrest needle and inject 5 ml of solution slowly. More often no paresthesias are met and then proceed to bone contact with humerus. Fan solution 2 to 3 cm proximally and distally to site of first bone contact, injecting 3 to 4 ml each time.
   (b) **At Wrist:** A 5-cm needle on a 10-ml syringe is advanced after cleansing and wealing of the skin. Radial-dorsal circumference of the hand is infiltrated with solution intradermally and subcutaneously. This is interrupted only if paresthesias (to thumb) are elicited. Then arrest needle and inject 1 to 2 ml of solution.

Evaluation of Effect: If paresthesias (to thumb or back of hand) were initiated, no skin testing is necessary. Otherwise use pin prick test.

Complications: None, unless aspiration was omitted; then, intravascular injection is possible.

Local Anesthetic: 5 to 10 ml of short- or long-acting drug. Sometimes adrenaline may be used.

Onset and Duration: After 2 to 5 (to 15) min effect lasts about 1 to 3 (3 to 8) hr. Solutions containing adrenaline act longer.

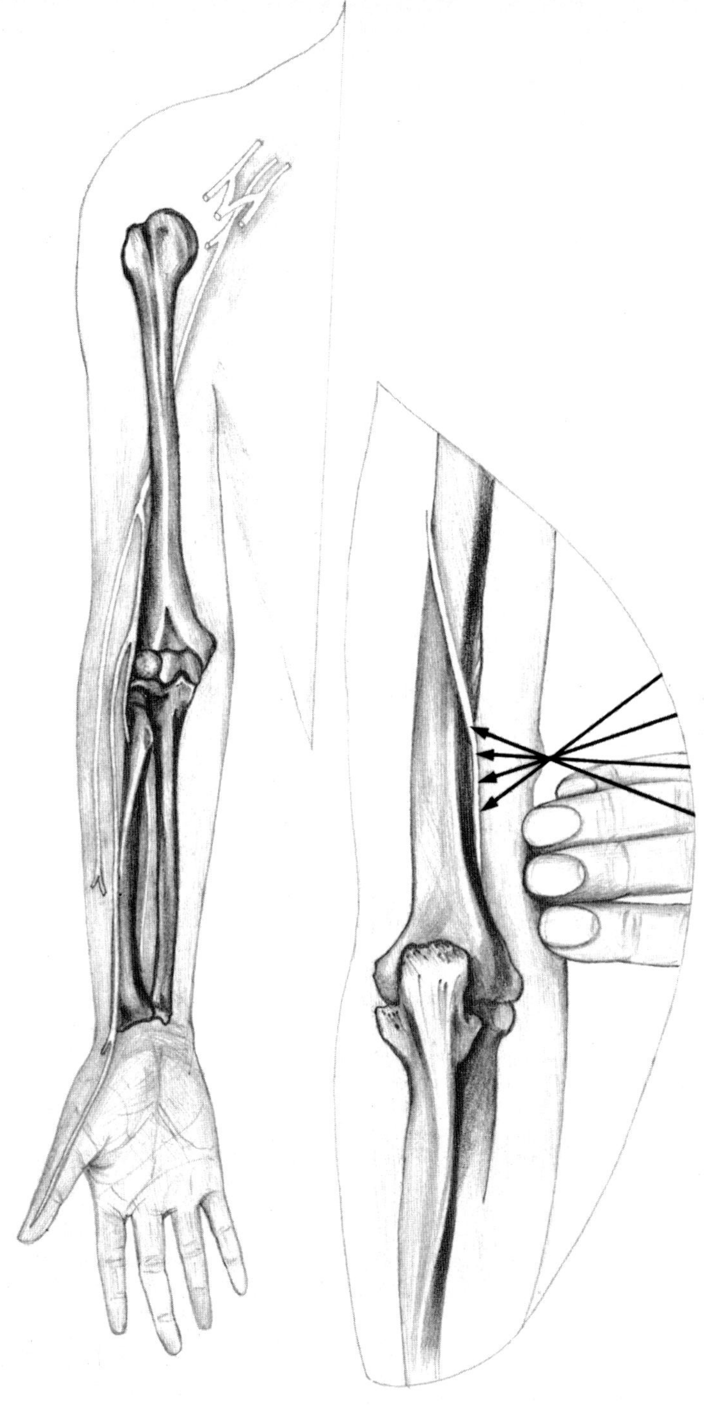

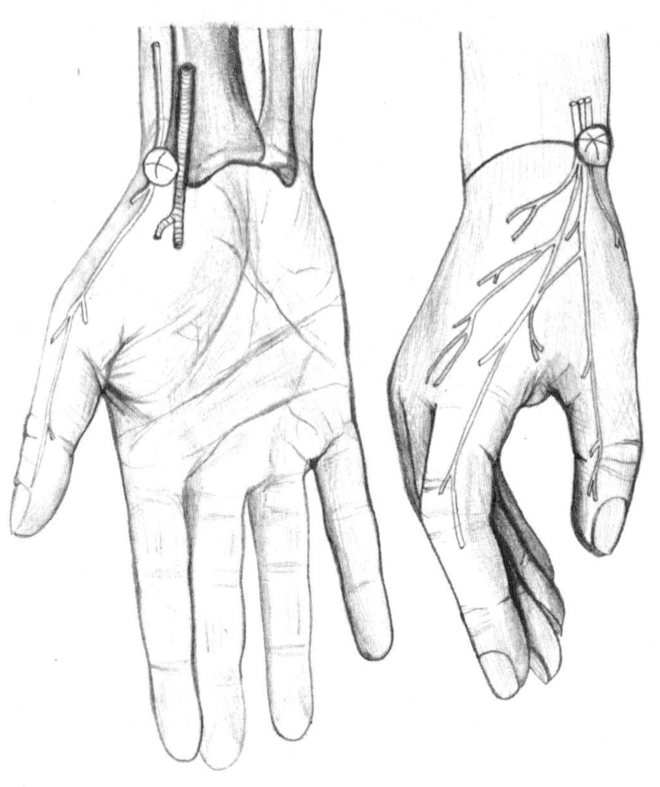

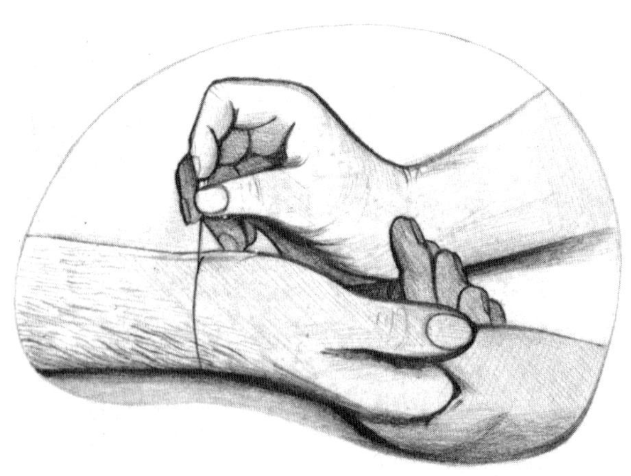

Suprascapular Nerve Block

Indications

1. **Diagnostic:** In localizing shoulder and upper back pain.
2. **Therapeutic:** Relief of pain, as in acute or chronic subacromial bursitis, humeroscapular periarthritis, together with physical therapy.
3. **Surgical:** None.

Technique

1. **Possibilities:** Two methods are described, differing mainly in the way to find the site of skin puncture.
2. **Position:** Sitting, arms crossed over abdomen. Also in the lateral position, having uppermost arm dropping over head end of examining table.
3. **Landmarks:** Through center of connecting line between scapular spine and tip of acromion, draw vertical (sagittal) line and line halving angle toward upper lateral quadrant of these two lines. 2 to 2.5 cm from point of intersection of lines, on halving line, mark skin.
4. **Point of Block:** Suprascapular nerve, as it leaves incision on cranial border of scapula to reach muscles on back of scapula.
5. **Procedure:** After skin cleansing and wealing at skin mark, an 8-cm needle with short bevel is advanced perpendicular to the skin, keeping a direction somewhat mediocaudally. After 3 to 7 cm, bone should be met. If this is not the case, one is justified in assuming that the needle point is placed in the incisure of the scapula, and 10 ml of solution are injected slowly. In case of bone contact, try to find the incision by moving the tip of the needle slightly and proceed as above.

Evaluation of Effect: Only rarely are paresthesias felt, because only in the unusual case is there a small sensory representation on the skin of the shoulder. Good blocking is characterized by default function of supraspinate and infraspinate muscles; i. e., there exists difficulty in abduction and outward rotation of upper arm. Also, subjectively, pain disappears.

Complications: None. If the needle is advanced deeper than indicated, there rarely occurs pneumothorax.

Local Anesthetic: 5 to 10 (3 to 8) ml of solution, without or with adrenaline.

Onset and Duration: After 2 to 5 (to 15) min. Block lasts for 2 to 3 (6 to 15) hr. This block is very suitable for relief of shoulder pain together with physical therapy.

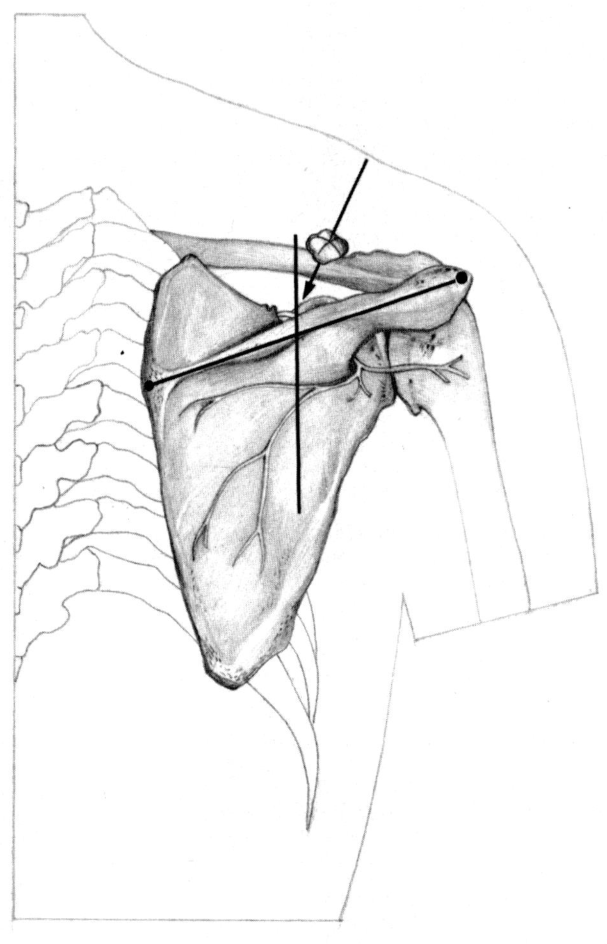

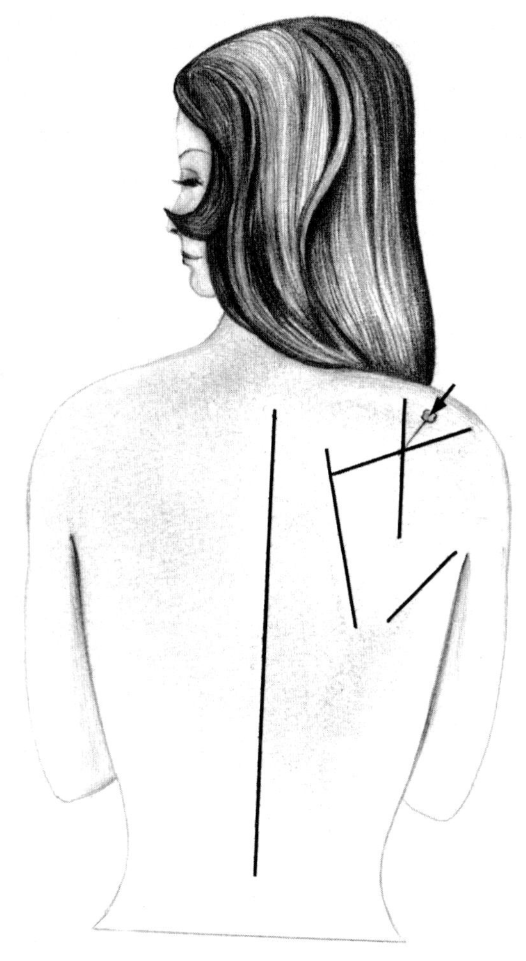

Intercostal Nerve Block

Indications

1. **Diagnostic:** In differentiating somatic from vegetative pain syndromes of the chest wall.

2. **Therapeutic:** Relief of pain following (serial) rib fractures, upper abdominal surgical procedures, here especially to further coughing and deep breathing as well as early ambulation and in cases of thoracic surgical procedures; postherpetic zoster neuralgias (in conjunction with sympathetic blocks), intercostal neuralgias of other origin, such as after surgical scars, pectoralis minor syndrome, lesions of chondro-costal junction. In treating painful states caused by primary malignancy (such as pulmonary neoplasms) or secondary lesions (metastatic lesions of vertebrae or ribs), it may help. But for these latter, paravertebral blocks of somatic nerve are advocated.

3. **Surgical:** None.

Technique

1. **Possibilities:**
   (a) Paravertebral at costal angle; this approach hits the entire nerve. It is best to inject some 6 to 7 cm (in case of lowest ribs up to 10) paramedially (line B of sketch on page 51).

   (b) 2 cm dorsomedially of posterior axillary line; advisable only if anterior branch is to be blocked (line A of sketch on page 51).
   (c) Anterior axillary line; only for distal third of rib and sternum, and finally,
   (d) Parasternally; suffices only for sternal fractures.

2. **Position:** Unilateral block requires lateral position of patient with diseased side (to be injected) up with arm held in a ventral-cranially extended fashion. Bilateral block requires prone position with pillow under chest. Both may be carried out in the sitting position; then, front of patient faces back of chair, with arms crossed over it.

3. **Landmarks:** Caudal margin of respective rib; either in a paramedian line or dorsomedial of the posterior axillary line.

4. **Point of Block:** Intercostal nerve in inferior sulcus of respective rib which is situated dorsocaudally of vessels (see figures on page 51).

5. **Procedure:** After cleansing and wealing (optional) of skin (the latter only after pulling skin over inferior margin of rib), a 2.5- to 3-cm needle is advanced through the weal into the bone contact. The needle should be filled with solution and on a 5-ml (for one segment) or 10-ml (for two or three segments) syringe and kept at an angle with the skin (caudally) of 80°. After reaching bone, withdraw the needle minimally and release skin traction. Let the needle tip slide over the rib margin. After losing bone contact, advance the needle some 0.2 or 0.3 cm, aspirate, and slowly inject 3 ml per nerve. Withdraw needle.

   Note: In very muscular individuals the latissimus dorsi muscle may prevent or make difficult the palpation of the ribs at the posterior axillary line. The same holds for the first three ribs, where the serratus anterior muscle prevents palpation of the ribs.

Complications: The only serious complication is pneumothorax and occurs only if the first step (palpation of the rib and reaching bone contact) is not exactly possible. No other complications.

Local Anesthetic: 3 ml of any solution per segment, without or with vasoconstrictor (adrenaline).

Onset and Duration: 2 (to 10) min to full effect, which lasts 2 to 3.5 (6 to 10) hr without adrenaline; with it duration is doubled.

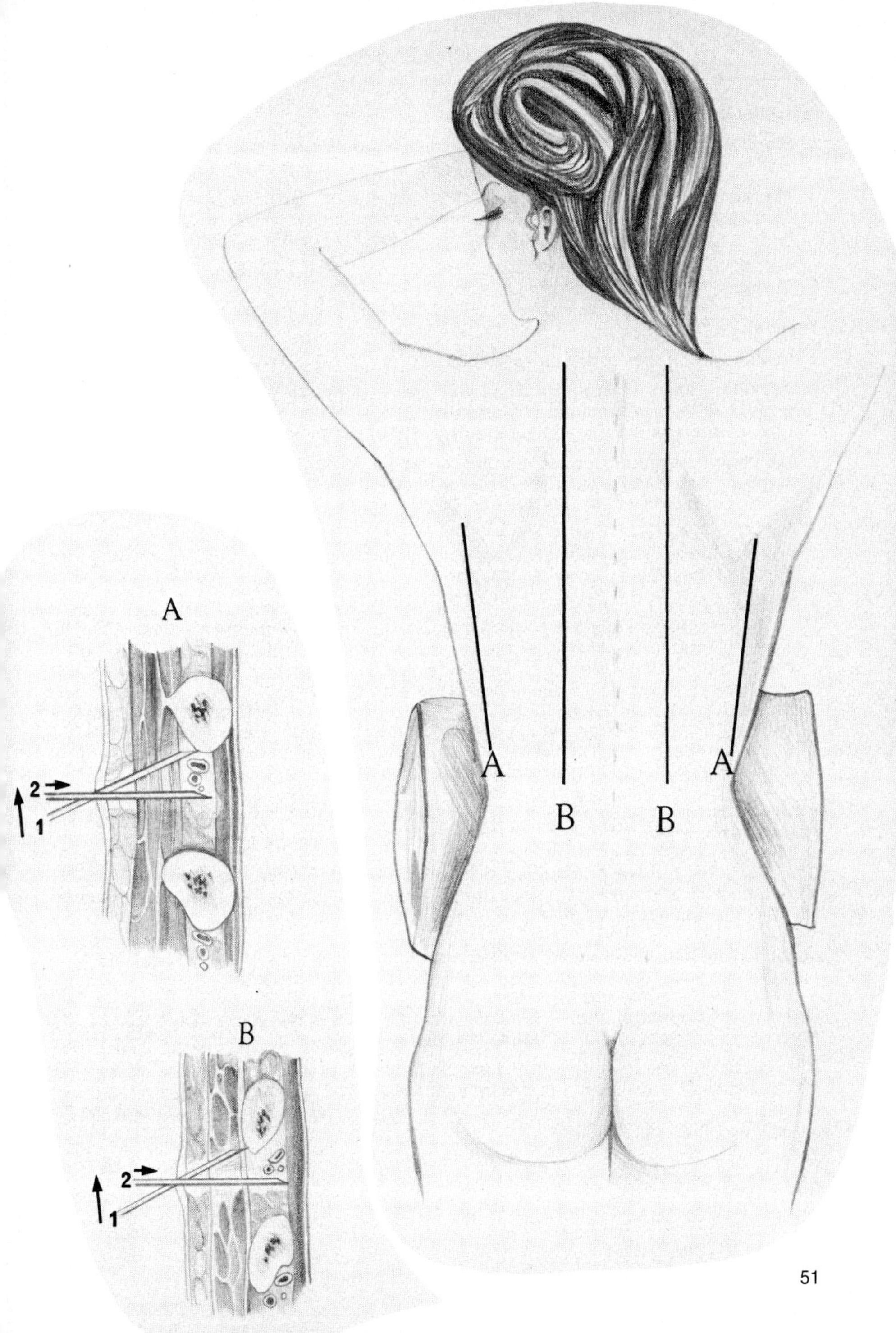
A
2
1
B
2
1
A
A
B
B

Paravertebral Thoracic Nerve Block

Indications

1. **Diagnostic:** In differentiating somatic from vegetative thoracic segmental and cardiac pain.
2. **Therapeutic:** Relief of pain in the intercostal area, such as postherpetic zoster neuralgia, causalgia; pain from primary (bronchial neoplasm) or secondary (vertebral or mediastinal metastases) malignant lesion. Postoperatively as in intercostal blocks (see there).
3. **Surgical:** None.

Technique

1. **Possibilities:** From dorsal paravertebrally.
2. **Position:** Patient in prone position with pillow under chest, no pillow under head. Arms dangle down both sides of examining table. When blocking first three nerves, it is advisable to have head hanging over end of examining table.
3. **Landmarks:** Through upper margins of dorsal spinous process of vertebra above segment that is to be blocked, draw (or imagine) a horizontal (transveral) line. Mark skin 4 cm lateral of midline on this line on side of block as point of insertion of needle.
4. **Point of Block:** Respective intercostal nerve immediately after it emerges from intervertebral foramen.
5. **Procedure:** After cleansing and wealing (optional) of skin at skin mark, an 8 (to 10)-cm needle is advanced perpendicular to the skin until bone contact is made with the transverse process of the respective vertebra. Mark depth of insertion on needle and withdraw needle to just beneath skin. Reinsert with tilt of 80° (cranially) to skin in a paramedian plane, barely passing below the transverse process, and proceed 2 to 2.5 cm deeper than the mark on the needle. When point of block is reached or paresthesias initiate aspirate (preferably with dry syringe) and inject 5 (to 10) ml of solution. It is desirable that during injection pain is either elicited or increased at painful site for which block is being made.

Evaluation: It is advantageous but not necessary to obtain paresthesias. If these are not observed, test with pin prick or rely on subjective disappearance of pain.

Complications: Subarachnoid injections may be possible when the needle point is directed medially and not kept in a paramedian plane. When the needle is pointing laterally, there is a faint possibility of pneumothorax. No other complications.

Local Anesthetic: Short-acting for diagnostic and long-acting for therapeutic block; in both instances, 5 (to 10) ml per segment, without or with adrenaline.

Onset and Duration: In 2 to 5 (10 to 15) min full effect is reached and will last 2 to 3.5 (4 to 12) hr. Longer duration is obtained with solutions containing adrenaline.

Remark: Paravertebral block of thoracic nerves is a simple and safe method, if all directions of procedure are strictly adhered to. The reaching of bone contact will give the proper depth; keeping the needle in a parasagittal plane will prevent the only possible complications.

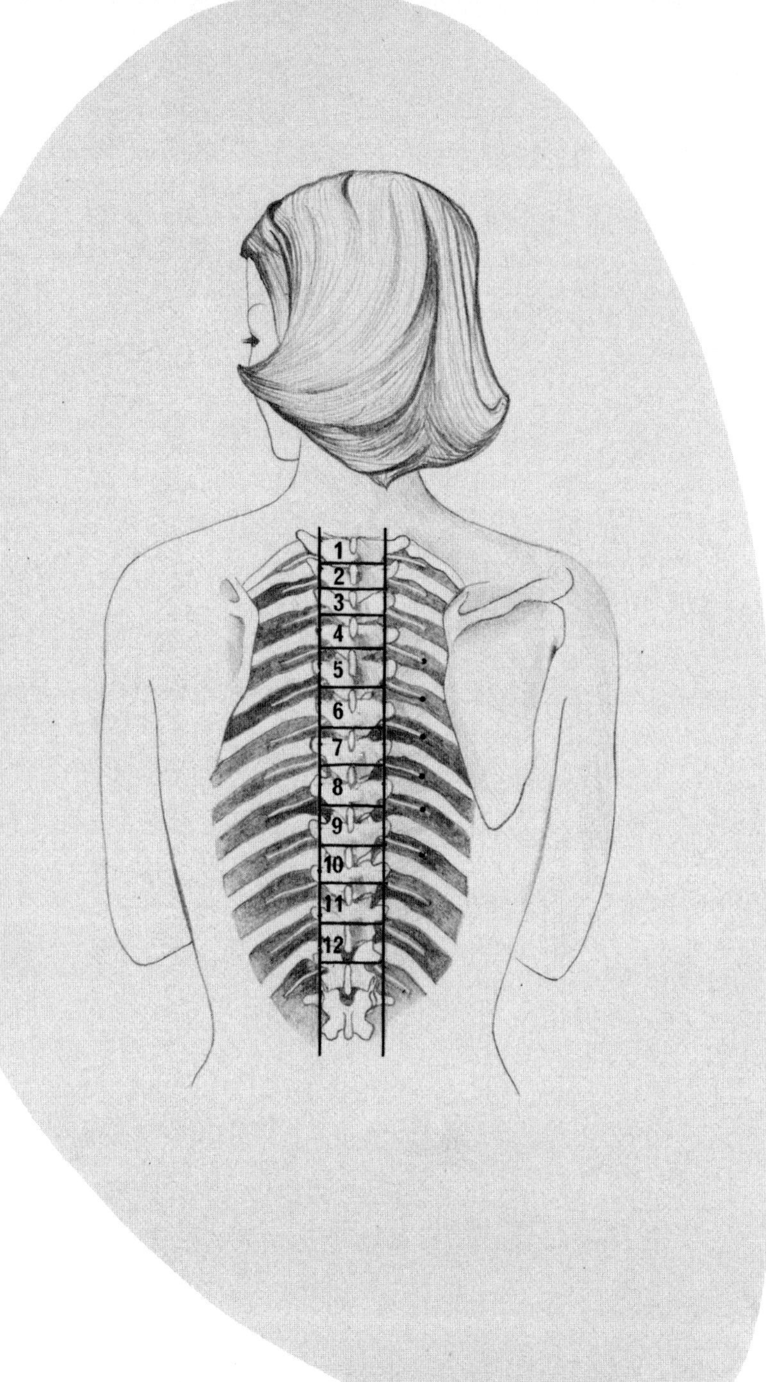
1
2
3
4
5
6
7
8
9
10
11
12

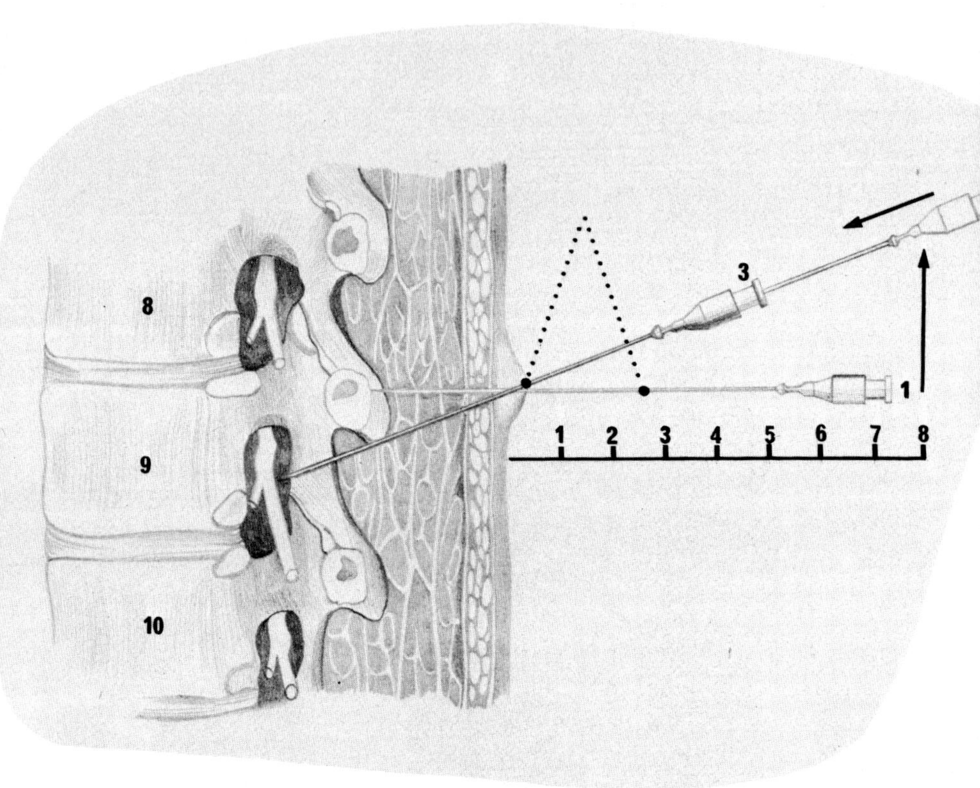

8
9
10
3
1
1
2
3
4
5
6
7
8

Paravertebral Lumbar Nerve Block

Indications

1. **Diagnostic:** To differentiate visceral pain in corresponding lower abdominal quadrant; to distinguish vascular disorders and somatic or vegetative pain conditions of leg.
2. Painful states of hip, kidney, inguinal regions, lateral, anterior and medial aspect of thigh; following lumbar vertebral fractures; meralgia paresthetica; segmental neuralgias such as may continue after laminotomy for protruded disk, spinal fusion, or with segmental involvement of either primary or secondary malignancies.
3. **Surgical:** None.

Technique

1. **Possibilities:** Paravertebral dorsal approach.
2. **Position:** Prone position with pillow under abdomen for bilateral block; or sitting with front facing back of chair and shoulders bent forward with arms folded around back of chair. Also lateral position with knees to chest for unilateral (upper) block.
3. **Landmarks:** Lowest point of dorsal spinous process of next (cranial) vertebra.
4. **Point of Block:** Spinal segmental lumbar nerve as it emerges from intervertebral foramen.
5. **Procedure:** After skin marking (3 to 4 cm lateral of lowest point of dorsal spinous process, see above), cleansing and wealing (optional), an 8 (to 10)-cm needle is advanced perpendicular to the skin surface until bone (of transverse process) is contacted. Mark depth of insertion of needle, withdraw needle to just beneath skin, and reinsert with a tilt of 80 to 85° caudally, barely passing the transverse process for 3 more cm (maximally). After 1.5 cm paresthesias may appear; if so, arrest needle. Then follows aspiration, injection of 5 (to 10) ml of solution, and withdrawal of needle.

Evaluation: Paresthesias indicate good needle position. Also, if during injection pain is increased, good placement of needle is ascertained. In other cases test with pin prick in respective segments 5 to 10 min after block or rely on subjective indications of disappearance of pain.

Complications: Usually none. Subarachnoid injection may rarely occur if the needle point is kept too far medially and not in a parasagittal plane. The loss of motor function in the blocked segment is not a complication but still surprises the patient. But because mixed nerves are blocked this should always be present and be regarded as positive evidence of exact placement of the block.

Local Anesthetic: For diagnostic purposes use short (fast)-acting drug, for therapeutic effects long-acting drug. (2 to 3 to) 5 ml usually suffice.

Onset and Duration: After 2 to 5 (to 10) min effect should be fully present and last about 2 to 3.5 (4 to 10) hr.

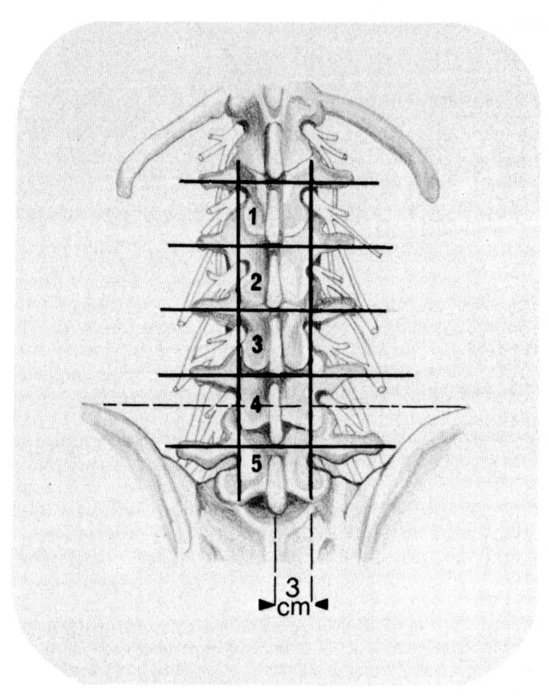
1
2
3
4
5
3
cm

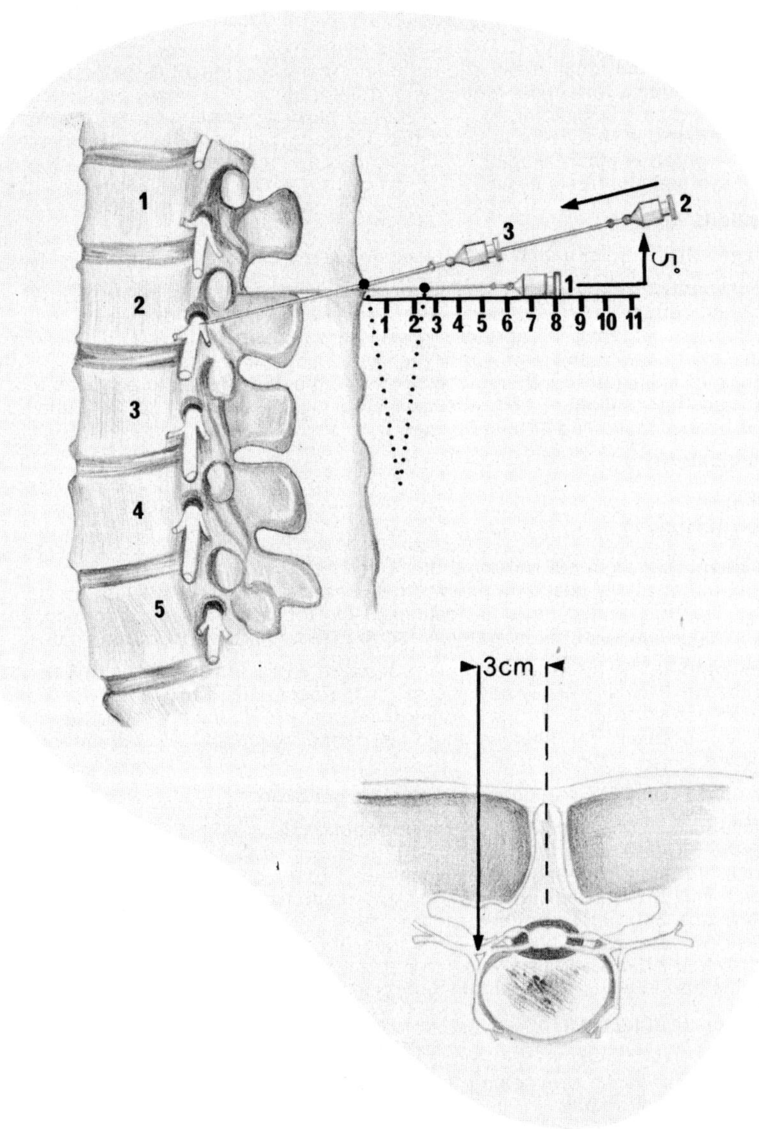
1
2
3
4
5
3
2
5°
1
1 2 3 4 5 6 7 8 9 10 11
3cm

Thoracic Sympathetic Block

Basic Remark: This block will be carried out rather seldom, because a stellate block will cover the sympathetic block of the segments thoracic 1 to 4 if ample solution is used (about 10 ml). Likewise, a splanchnic or high lumbar sympathetic block will cover the thoracic segments 6 to 12. These facts have been proven by admixing contrast X-ray medium to the local anesthetic solution. Therefore, thoracic sympathetic block is reserved for those rare cases where sympathetic block of a single segment is wanted. Should there be no objection to simultaneous block of somatic spinal nerves and sympathetic fibers, it should be recalled that blocking paravertebrally the somatic spinal nerves – which is much simpler – will also reach communicant rami and therefore interrupt sympathetic fibers as well as somatic.

Indications

1. **Diagnostic:** Differentiating cardiac and epigastric pain.
2. **Therapeutic:** In cases of angina pectoris, sympathogenic disorders of cardiac rhythm, asthma, pulmonary embolism, esophageal pain, cardiospasm, together with somatic nerve block in cases of thoracic herpes zoster neuralgia, gall bladder or renal colics, pancreatic pain, paralytic ileus, megacolon, cardiospasm; for hyperhidrosis of axilla either a thoracic sympathetic block or a stellate ganglion block is indicated. For malignant pain alternate blocking of somatic and sympathetic nerves has been advised and should be tried.
3. **Surgical:** None.

Technique

1. **Possibilities:** Form paravertebral dorsal only.
2. **Position:** Just as in paravertebral block of thoracic somatic spinal nerves prone position, pillow under chest, no pillow under head. Also occasionally in the sitting position, but then patient must be placed in the recumbent position immediately after blocking because of fall in systemic blood pressure after sympathetic block.
3. **Landmarks:** The tip of the spinous process of thoracic vertebrae 4 to 8 corresponds to the next lower transverse process. In the segments 1 to 3 and 6 to 12 the tip of the spines correspond to the intervertebral space, i. e., the space between the transverse processes. The needle should pierce the skin about 4 (to 6) cm lateral of the midline.
4. **Point of Block:** The respective sympathetic ganglion.
5. **Procedure:** After cleansing and wealing (optional) of skin at proper site, a 5 to 8-cm needle on a 10 ml syringe, both filled, is advanced to bone contact with the transverse process. The needle is then marked 1 to 1.5 cm over skin level, withdrawn to just beneath the skin, and reinserted in a plane tilted 10° cranially of the transverse plane and 30° medially of the sagittal plane, barely sliding over the edge of transverse process. There should be constant bone contact. On the ventral face of the transverse process and rib, meaning at the moment of loss of bone contact, arrest needle and inject 5 (to 10) ml of solution slowly (no sketch).

Evaluation of Effect: There will be subjective loss of pain; when blocking one or two segments only, there is no other control possible.

Complications: When proceeding too far beyond transverse processes or rib, there is danger of pneumothorax.

Local Anesthetic: 5 to 10 ml of fast-acting or 3 to 5 ml of long-acting drug; never use adrenaline or other vasoconstrictors.

Onset and Duration: After 2 to 5 (10 to 20) min full effect should be reached and will last about 2 to 3 (6 to 12) hr.

Lumbar Sympathetic Block

Indications

1. **Diagnostic:** In differentiating various pain problems and vascular disorders of the lower extremity. To prognosticate the possible effect of surgical section of lumbar sympathetic chain.
2. **Therapeutic:** In relief of various painful states of the lower extremity such as pain from vascular (arterial) insufficiency, arterial embolism, thrombosis, aneurysms, Raynaud's disease, Buerger-Winiwarters' disease, all peripheral vascular disorders accompanied by vasospastic component; postphlebitic edema, contractures following plaster casts, cold trauma, posttraumatic dystrophies of bone and osteoporosis, phantom pain, causalgias; as supplementary therapy in chronic infectious processes of lower extremities, badly healing leg ulcers, hyperhidrosis of lower half of body, articular stiffness. In relieving pain from acute and subacute pancreatitis, arthritis, muscle spasm, and as a trial in Hirschsprung's disease and megacolon.
3. **Surgical:** None.

Technique

1. **Possibilities:** From paravertebral dorsal only.
2. **Position:** Lateral position, knees to chest; rarely prone position. May also be carried out in the sitting position, but patient must be placed horizontal immediately after block (see complications: fall in blood pressure).
3. **Landmarks:** From mid of dorsal spinous process of respective vertebra, a transversal line is drawn on which at 9 cm distance from the sagittal plane the needle is inserted.
4. **Point of Block:** Sympathetic ganglion of respective vertebra, on antero-lateral aspect of vertebral body.
5. **Procedure:** After cleansing and wealing (optional) of skin, a 10- to 12- to 15-cm needle is inserted at the skin mark in a parasagittal plane, directed cranially, 80° angle to skin caudally, until bone contact with transverse process of same vertebra is made. Mark depth of needle and withdraw halfway. Reinsert in a transverse plane, tip directed slightly medially, at an angle to the skin of 85° laterally. Advance needle 4 to 4.5 cm more than before with bevel pointing medially. Ideally, periosteal or bone contact is barely made. Just after this is lost, i. e., maximally 4.5 cm deeper than transverse process, aspirate and inject 10 to 15 ml of local anesthetic. Remove syringe and inject 1 ml of air to prevent local anesthetic from reaching spinal nerve and withdraw needle.

Complications: It is advisable to use rather thin (0.8 mm diameter) needles to circumvent bleeding; when slowly injecting solution while advancing needle, this will not occur. The only noteworthy complication is disproportional fall of blood pressure. For this reason it should be strictly observed that patients stay in a horizontal position from 15 to about 45 min after block, depending on case and reaction of blood pressure. Blood pressure should be controlled initially about q. 5 min. Inadvertant block of spinal (lumbar segmental) nerve is unimportant.

Local Anesthetic: Short- or long-acting drugs, 10 to 15 ml; may occasionally be done with 96 percent alcohol.

Onset and Duration: Signs of onset are vasodilatation and increase of skin temperature in legs. Both appear about 5 to 10 (to 15) min after blocking and should last about 3 hr (6 to 15 hr). A series of daily blocks may have a prolonged effect for up to several months.

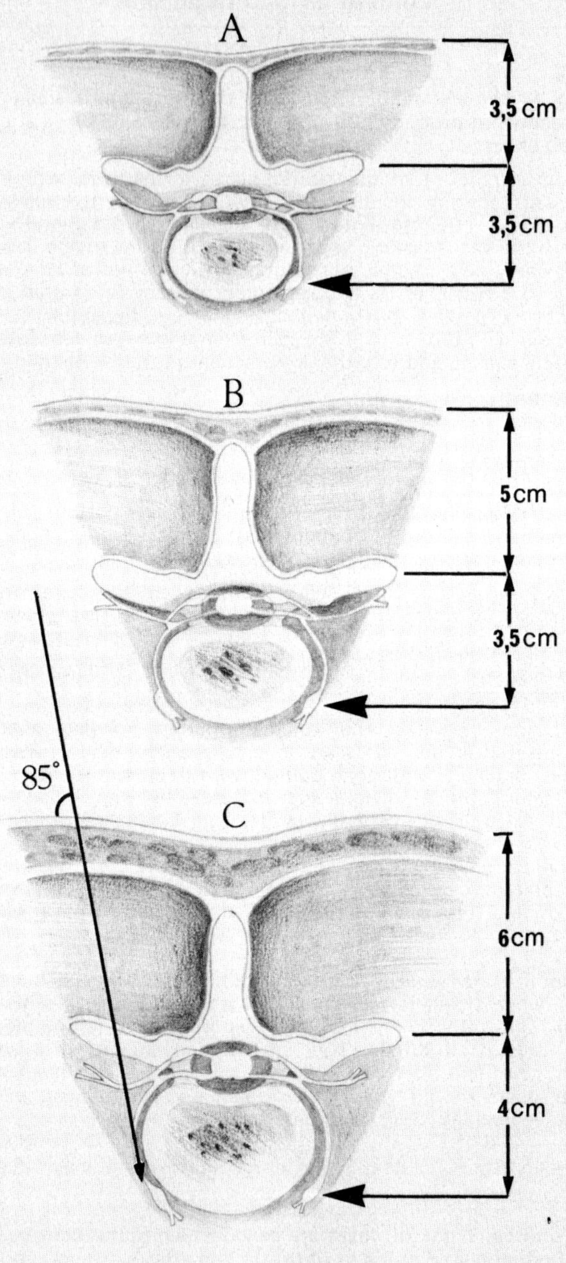

A
3,5 cm
3,5 cm
B
5 cm
3,5 cm
85°
C
6 cm
4 cm

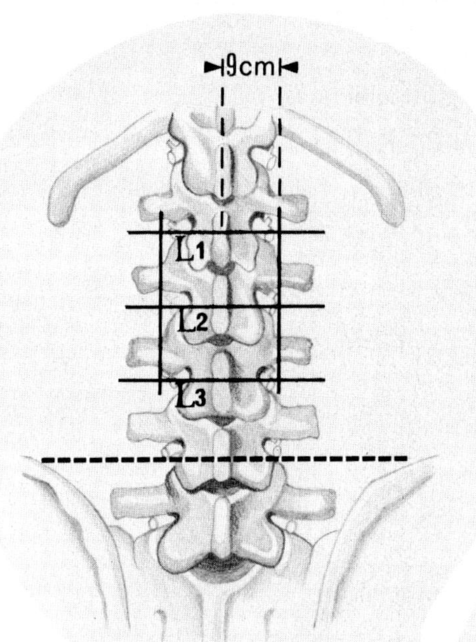
9cm
L1
L2
L3

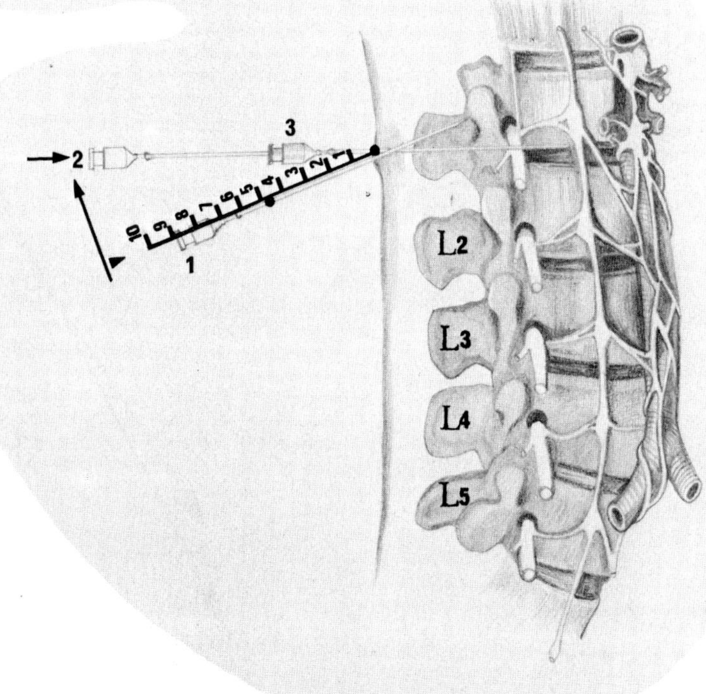
3
2
1
10
9
8
7
6
5
4
3
2
1
L2
L3
L4
L5

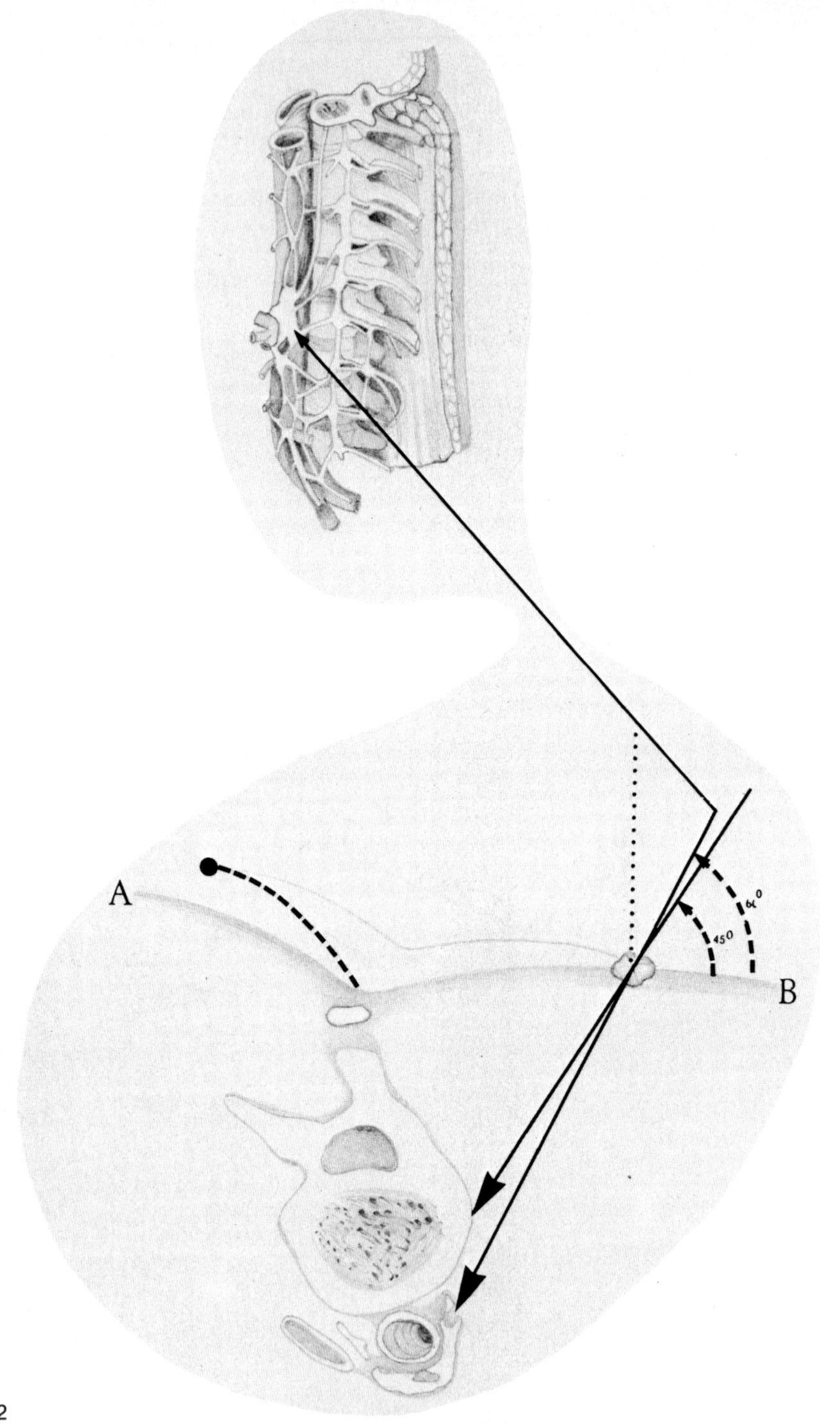
A
B
45°
60°

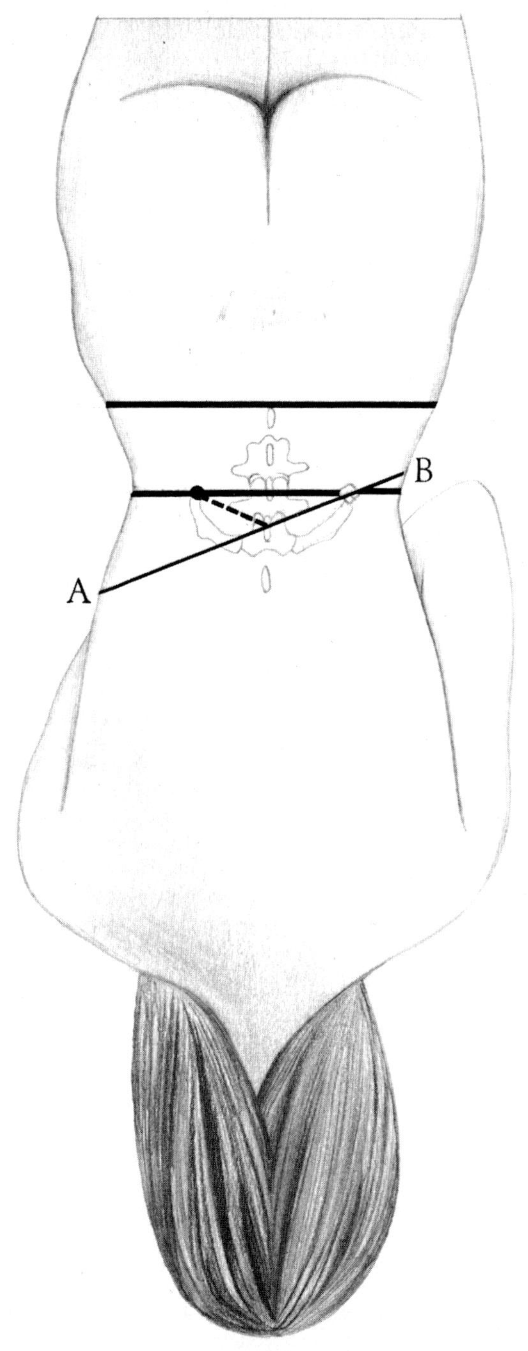
B
A

Splanchnic (Celiac Ganglion) Block

Indications

1. **Diagnostic:** In differentiating visceral from abdominal wall pain and from cardiac pain.
2. **Therapeutic:** Relief of abdomino-visceral pain, e. g., from pancreas. Sometimes, influencing dumping symdrome. In cases of septic, traumatic, and hemorrhagic shock to counteract vasospasm in splanchnic and renal vascular areas (occasionally this may obtain vital importance). Peptic ulcer, paralytic ileus.
3. **Surgical:** As supportive measure in cases where operations on upper abdomen are carried out under local anesthesia.

Technique

1. **Possibilities:** Percutaneously from dorsal; otherwise from open abdomen.
2. **Position:** Prone position, pillow under abdomen between costal margin and iliac crests.
3. **Landmarks:** Connecting line between iliac crests meets the space between third and fourth lumbar spinous process or the fourth spine. From here locate dorsal spinous processes of twelfth thoracic and first lumbar vertebrae. Control by counting down from first thoracic spine. Mark both spines. Now palpate twelfth rib bilaterally 6 to 8 cm from midline (depending on constitution of patient: lateral margin of sacrospinal muscle) and mark skin there. Between these three skin marks, there is usually formed a triangle with very low height (see sketch).
4. **Point of Block:** Celiac ganglion situated in paravertebral space anterior to cranial (upper) anterior margin of first lumbar vertebral body bilaterally.
5. **Procedure:** After cleansing and wealing of skin at left costal mark, affix a 12- to 15 cm needle onto a filled 20 ml syringe and fill needle with solution. Now advance needle through weal in a direction pointing to lower border of twelfth thoracic spinous process tilted to the skin in a 45° angle laterally open until bone (= body of first lumbar vertebra) is contacted. Depth of needle is marked and needle withdrawn halfway. Now insert at 60° angle to skin surface and pass first lumbar vertebral body by 1 to 1.5 cm. Needle should barely touch bone or periosteum. In this new depth aspirate and inject 20 to 25 ml of local anesthetic.

Evaluation of Effect: Peritoneum and viscera (not in small pelvis) are anesthetized.

Complications: Pneumothorax (rarely) and fall in blood pressure (rather frequently observed) follow the block. Therefore, patients should rest in a reclining position for 1 hr after the block. As a precaution, it is advised that patients (1) have an empty stomach and (2) do not suppress coughing; when patient coughs, interrupt injection immediately.

Remark: In looking at the sketch on page 62 it becomes evident that puncturing of or passing the needle through various intraabdominal organs becomes not only possible but necessary. The literature mentions no sequelae of such microtraumatism such as hematuria peritonitis, or the like, even though more than 3,000 - cases had been followed rather closely. One is correct in assuming that these punctures must either be followed by very minimal or no traumatism at all. In any event it is advised that the celiac ganglion be blocked only if the patient is not in poor condition.

Local Anesthetic: 20 to 25 ml of any drug, mostly very weak solutions, such as 0.5 percent lidocaine; if using more potent drugs such as bupivacaine, the 0.25 percent solution has to be diluted 1 : 1 with 0.9 percent NaCl to be suitable.

Onset and Duration: 5 to 10 (to 20) min after block effect should be manifest and should last about 1.5 to 3 (3 to 6) hr.

Transsacral Nerve Block

Indications

1. **Diagnostic:** In differentiating pain problems of lower extremities and the perineal and perianal region.
2. **Therapeutic:** Relief of pain in the named area; in supporting relief of pain in malignant disease of pelvic area, in which case 96 percent alcohol may be used as the blocking agent. To relieve sphincter spasm of bladder in cases of spinal cord injury when sufficient muscular tone is ascertained cystometrographically.
3. **Surgical:** None. But in principle, operations on hemorrhoids or a coccygectomy would be possible.

Technique

1. **Approach:** Through sacral foramina.
2. **Position:** Prone position, one or two pillows under iliac crest, legs slightly spread, toes turned inward, heels outward to achieve relaxation of gluteal muscles.
3. **Landmarks:** Sacral cornua are palpated and marked, as are the posterior superior iliac spines. The dorsal openings of the second sacral foramina are situated 1 to 1.5 cm medial and caudal of the spines. The dorsal openings of the fourth sacral foramina may be felt 1 cm cephalad and lateral of the sacral cornua. Connections of these points should be parallel to each other and the midsagittal line. The first foramen may be felt 2 cm above the second foramen and somewhat more laterally. The fifth sacral nerve turns around the cornu 2 cm caudal of the fourth foramen; the third sacral foramen lies between the second and fourth somewhat closer to the second.
4. **Point of Block:** Sacral nerves in the respective sacral foramina. Note: The direction of the canals is from cranial to medio-caudal. Asymmetries of the foramina are quite common.
5. **Procedure:** A 2 × 2 is inserted into the anal fold to prevent prepping solution from reaching the mucous membranes. After cleansing and wealing the skin over the respective foramen, an 8-cm needle is advanced through the skin. For the fourth and fifth foramen, a 5-cm needle is sufficient. For the second nerve, a 10-cm needle may be required. The needle is passed through the sacral foramen (after palpating its border with the needle point) 1.5 to 2 cm. In case of paresthesias the needle is arrested immediately. 5 to 10 ml of the chosen solution are injected. While removing the needle some milliliters of the solution are injected. It may be advisable to palpate the dorsal opening of the foramen once more with the needle point.

Evaluation: The effect appears as paresthesias relatively frequently. Analgesia in the corresponding segments may be checked with a needle point.

Complications: Practically none are observed if aspiration is performed correctly before the injection. If not, intravascular and intrathecal injections may occur. The block is carried out more easily if due attention is paid to the frequent occurrence of asymmetries when marking the skin.

Local Anesthetic: Lidocaine or mepivacaine, 1 to 2 percent, 5 to 10 ml. For longer action, 0.5 percent 2 ml or 0.25 percent, 3 to 5 ml bupivacaine per nerve. Strictly observe maximum dose when injecting more segments. In cases of malignancy 96 percent alcohol may be used.

Onset and Duration: Shorter-acting drugs: After 5 to 10 min for 1 and 1/2 to 2 1/2 hr, the longer-acting drugs after 10 to 20 min for 5 to 12 hr or longer, depending on solutions with or without adrenaline.

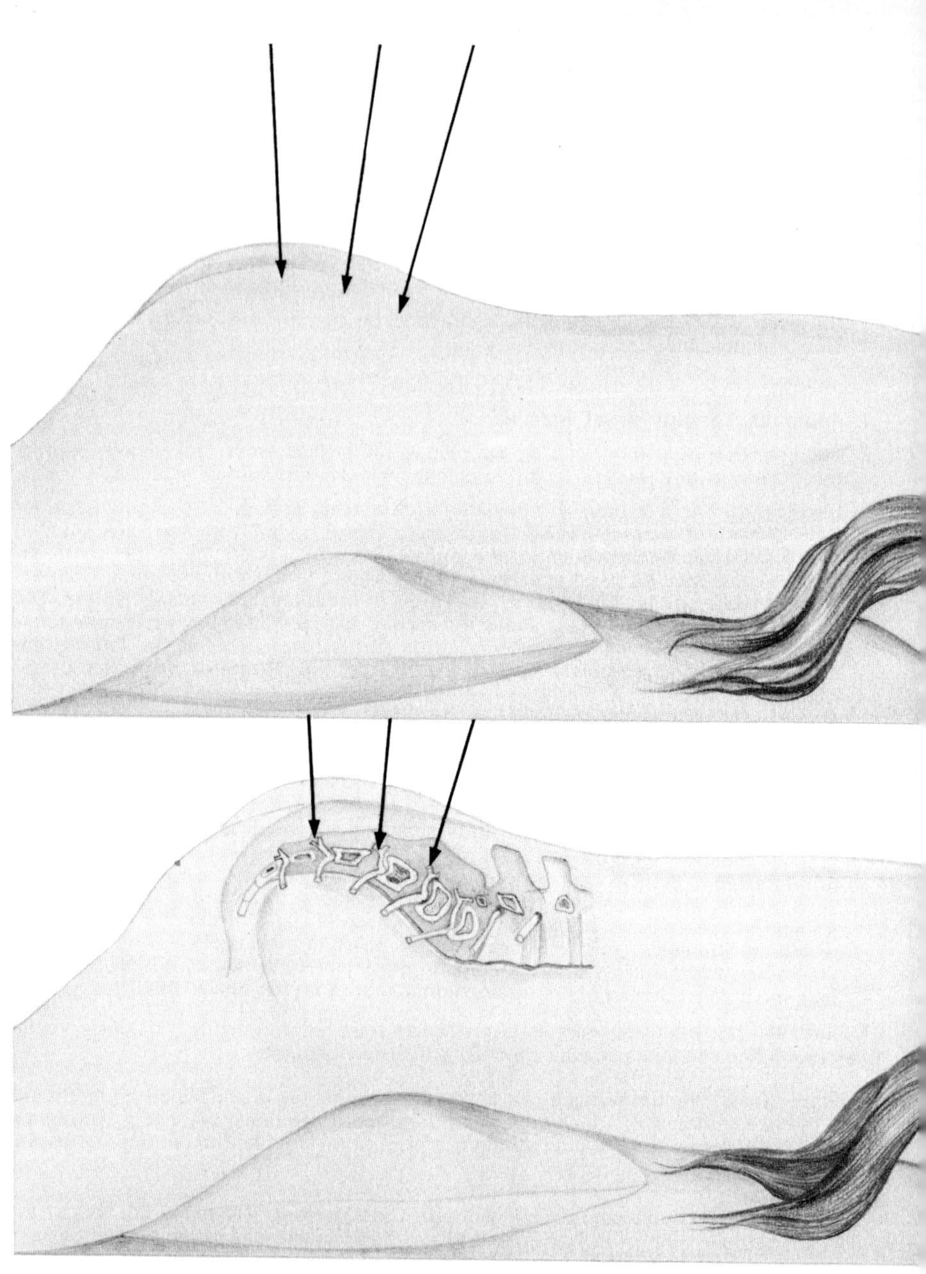

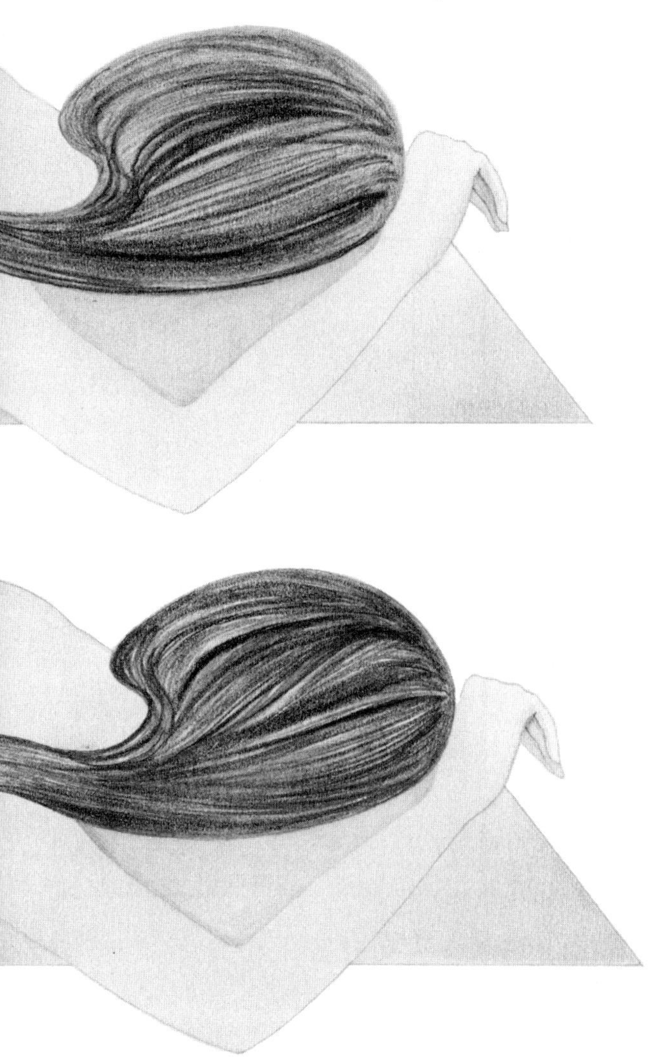

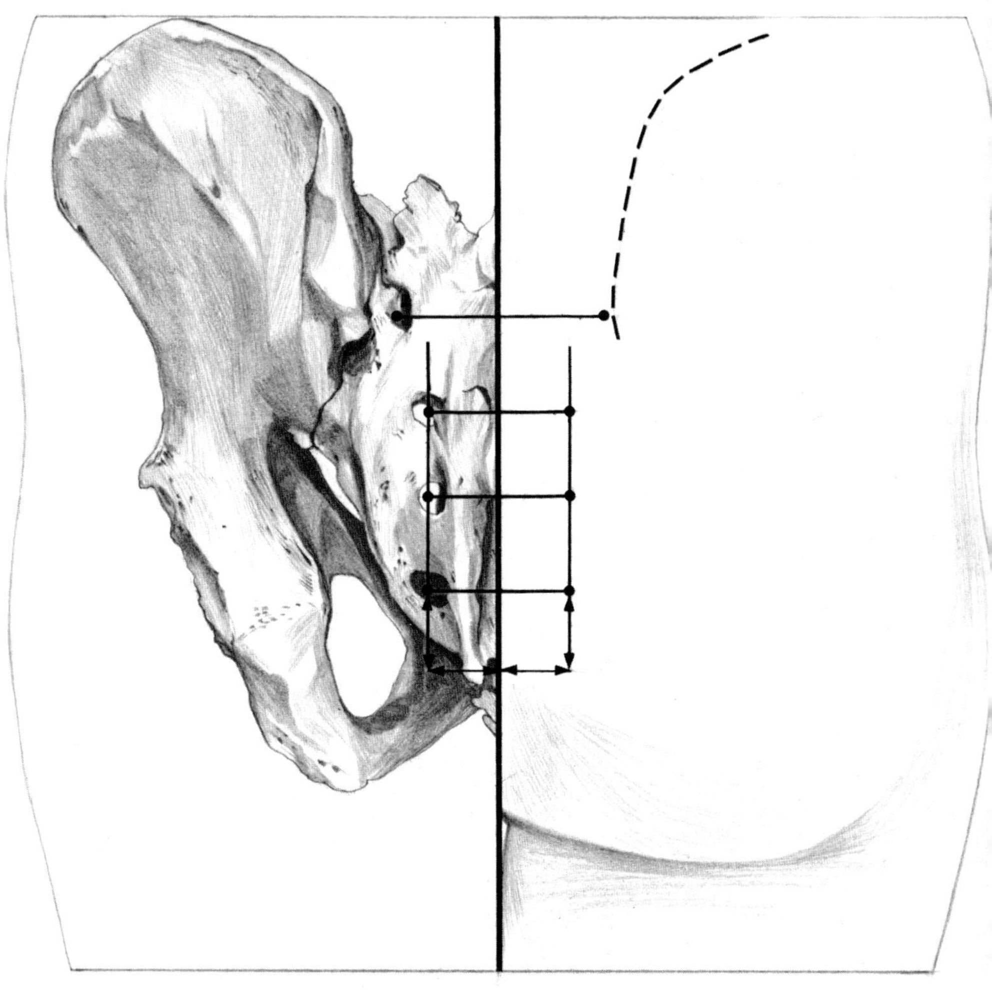

Pudendal Block

Indications

1. **Diagnostic:** Rarely for differentiating perianal pain.
2. **Therapeutic:** Occasionally for alleviation of pain in terminal stage of malignant disease of vulva of perineal pain.
3. **Obstetric:** This is the main indication: Pain relief during second stage of normal uncomplicated labor. Always bilaterally.

Technique

1. **Possibilities:**
   (a) **Percutaneously** and
   (b) **Transvaginally.**
2. **Position:** Lithotomy position, restraint.
3. **Landmarks:** Tuberosity of ischium, where pudendal nerve passes by (see sketch).
4. **Point of Block:** Pudendal nerve, as it passes ischial tuberosity.
5. **Procedure:**
   (a) **Percutaneously:** After cleansing and wealing of skin over tuberosity of ischium, insert gloved finger of left hand (in case of right-handed operator) into rectum or vagina and palpate tuberosity. The palpating finger stays in place during the entire procedure. Now insert a 6- to 8-cm needle on a filled 10-ml syringe to bone (about 2.5 to 4 cm), aspirate, and inject slowly under control of index finger 8 to 10 ml of solution around tuberosity. Then withdraw needle and remove finger.
   (b) **Transvaginally:** Prepare vagina with Phisohex or the like. The guide with the injecting needle (Kobak needle, Bofors needle, Iowa trumpet; with ball tip) fixed is introduced into the vagina between the index and middle fingers of the right hand (in right-handed examiner and normal vaginal examining position of hand) and ball brought close to ischial tuberosity. Palpation of this is easy through soft parts. Now disengage fixation of injecting needle and advance it 1.5 cm (no more possible) after setting a filled 10 ml syringe on it. After aspiration inject slowly 8 to 10 ml per side onto tuberosity. Then withdraw needle with guide and hand.

Evaluation: Paresthesias are extremely rare and not sought.

Complications: None.

Local Anesthetic: 8 to 10 ml per side. Block usually is done bilaterally. In case of long-acting drug beware of single maximum dose.

Onset and Duration: Immediate onset; 0.5 to 2 (1 to 3,5) hr duration.

Remark: For other than obstetric block transsacral or epidural (caudal) block is preferred as the resulting anesthesia is more satisfactory and the procedure less time consuming.

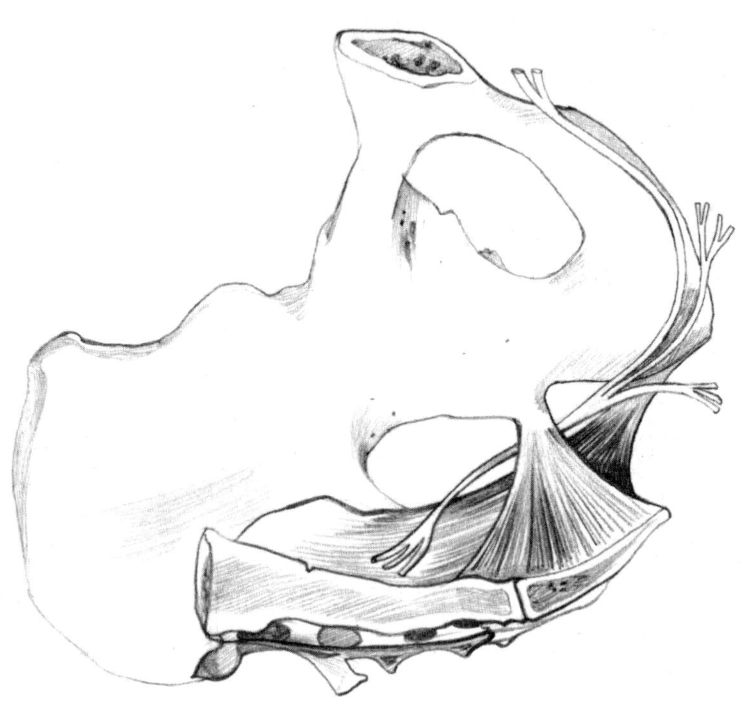

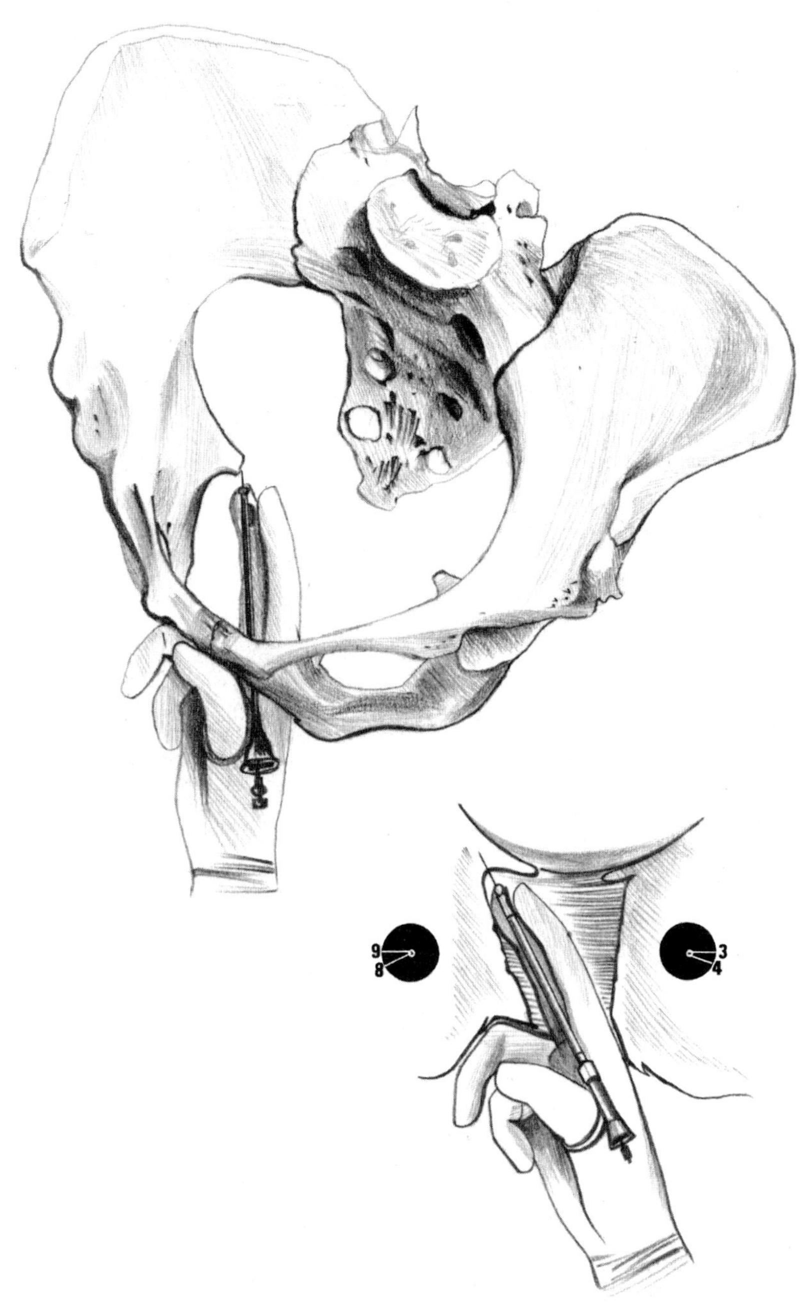
9
8
3
4

Paracervical (Uterosacral) Block

Indications

1. **Obstetrical:** Main indication; alleviates pain during first stage of normal, uncomplicated labor.
2. **Gynecological:** For small procedures on portio of cervix (by some); also for curettage.

Technique

1. **Possibility:** Transvaginally.
2. **Position:** Supine, legs spread apart and in partial lithotomy position.
3. **Landmarks:** At between 3 and 4 and 8 and 9 o'clock on lateral fornix of vagina.
4. **Point of Block:** Frankenhäuser's ganglion.
5. **Procedure:** Wait until cervix has a diameter of 5 cm (in case of a primipara) or 4 cm for a multipara (if good and forceful contractions are present, even 3 cm). Prepare vagina with Phisohex or the like. Between two pains, a guide with a fixed needle is introduced. This may be a Kobak needle, Bofors needle, or Iowa trumpet. In the latter case, affix syringe before introducing the instrument. When an instrument with bayonet-type connectors is used (such as B and D), affix syringe before disengaging fixation of needle. After instrument is in place, injecting canula is disenganged and advanced 1 to 1.5 cm through the ligament. After aspiration, 5 to 10 ml are injected per side. After blocking one side, it is advised to let two pains pass before blocking second side.

Evaluation: Most frequently, the contraction following the block is not felt as painful on the side of block.

Complications: Various authors observed with changing percentile fetal bradycardia and in some rare cases also changes in fetal blood pH. The reasons for this have not been elucidated. Because of this, a typical case of high risk should therefore not be handled by paracervical block. It is also advised to exclude prophylactically the following cases from this type of "painless" labor: restless women, history of epileptiform or preeclamptic states, and amnionitis.

Local Anesthetic: Any short-acting solution in 1 percent concentration and the long-acting bupivacaine only in the lower concentration of 0.25 percent. Most authors prefer not to use adrenaline, but some also use solutions with adrenaline for this obstetrical indication.

Onset and Duration: Almost immediate onset is followed by full effect of only 0.5 to 2 hr (1.5 to 3.5) on the average, because of richness of blood supply to the injected site.

Remark: Combined with pudendal block, it reliefes pain of first and second stage of labor. Most recently, the injection is not done into the fornix but into the wall of the cervical canal itself. More experience on this type of injection, however, is still lacking.

Epidural (Caudal) Block

Indications

1. **Diagnostic:** In differentiating lumbar, coccygeal, or ischialgic pain.
2. **Therapeutic:** Alleviation of pain of vasospastic and organic nature in the distribution of the sacral nerves.
3. **Surgical:** For painless conduction of surgical procedures or operations on anus, rectum, or sigmoid, prostate, ureter, urethra, external genitalia, and in obstetrics. Continuous caudal anesthesia occasionally is still used in obstetrics because in these cases extremely long periods of analgesia are desirable. But the use of tubes placed epidurally has decreased markedly since the advent of extremely long-acting local anesthetics.

Technique

1. **Possibilities:** Via sacral canal.
2. **Position:** Prone position with pillow under pelvis.
3. **Landmarks:** Sacral cornua and os coccygis mark the corners of a triangle through which the sacral canal is easily reached.
4. **Point of Block:** Epidural space within the sacral canal.
5. **Procedure:** After cleansing and wealing skin, an 8 (to 10)-cm needle is pierced through the skin exactly at midline, between sacral cornua. Infiltrating slowly, the needle is advanced through the subcutis and periosteum into the sacral canal. If this is reached, replace syringe by one filled with air and inject 1 to 2 ml of air while a fingertip is placed on the skin exactly over the supposed position of the needle tip. If air (in the form of skin emphysema) is felt, withdraw needle and reinsert properly. If no air is palpated, replace syringe by one with local anesthetic and slowly inject and advance needle until maximally to the level of the second sacral foramina (see transsacral block). Aspiration in various directions is done and if no blood or CSF is obtained, inject 1 ml of anesthetic in 2 sec until the desired amount, usually between 15 and 30 ml, has been injected. Withdraw needle, injecting another 5 ml on the way out. Place patient in supine position. If clear fluid (= CSF) has been aspirated, the decision has to be made whether it is desirable to continue the procedure as a low spinal anesthesia (which is possible) or discontinue the block and choose some other means of pain relief outside the sacral canal. If blood has been aspirated, withdraw needle and reinsert in a slightly different position so that on aspiration no blood is obtained.

Evaluation: Check sensation with needle prick. Mostly, between twelfth thoracic dermatome and toes, analgesia of thighs and legs is found, more complete and persistant on ventral face, if patient has been placed too long in prone position, more complete on dorsal aspect, if patient was placed in supine position immediately after blocking. Should analgesia be desired on one side only, patient has to be placed on that side immediately after removing needle.

Complications: If carried out properly, intrathecal injection should not occur. Urine retention may occur after caudal block for various lengths of time and may require catheterization once or twice before resolving. Among the various nerve blocking procedures, breaking of needles is seen more often in this than in any other block. Should a needle break, go ahead and remove the fragment immediately, if necessary by surgery.

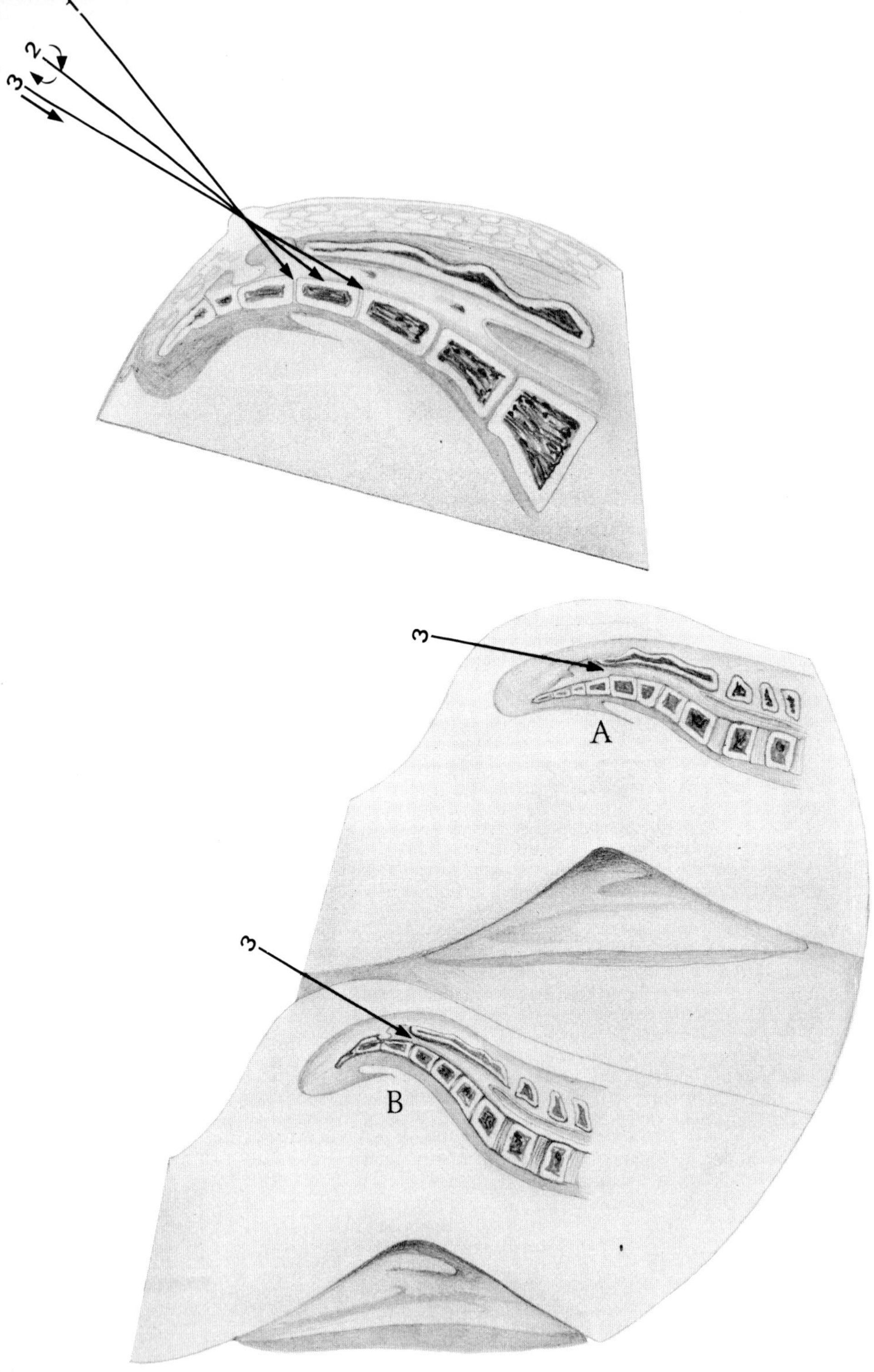
1
2
3
3
A
3
B

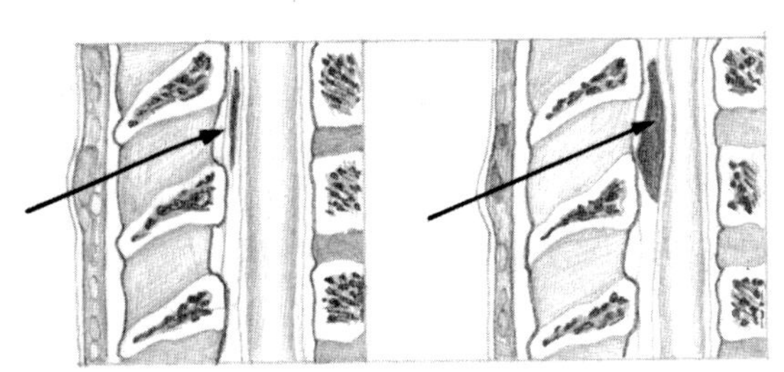

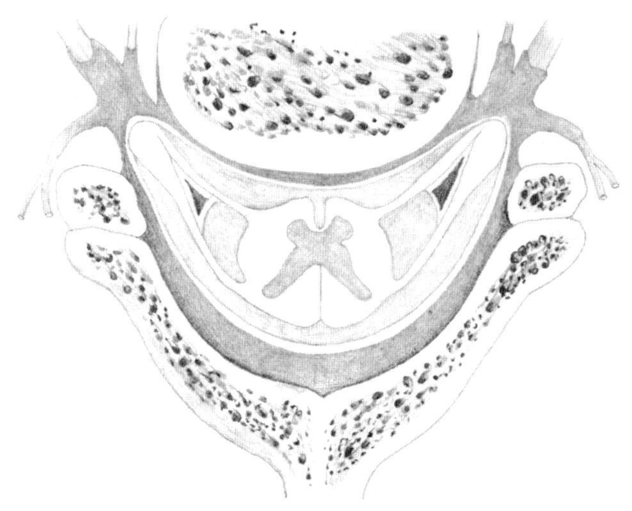

Local Anesthetic: 15 to 30 ml of any shorter-acting anesthetic, or up to 20 ml of a long-acting drug, mostly with adrenaline 1:200,000. If only a sympathetic block is desired, use lowest concentration of any anesthetic (e. g., 0.5 percent lidocaine) and no motor paresis will be seen. However, one should always remember that the volume of the peridural space varies greatly and so does the amount of fatty tissue present in this space. The level of analgesia and its depth will depend on these two factors. It is therefore understood that the level achieved is a matter of experience in judging the volume of the epidural space free of fat and difficult to prognosticate. As a guide, the average quantities of local anesthetic for various heights of levels of analgesia are as follows:

Saddle block	10 ml	To thoracic 6	40 ml
To lumbar 3	20 ml	To thoracic 3/4	50 ml
To thoracic 10	30 ml		

Onset and Duration: 3 to 5 min after injection, skin temperature (subjectively and objectively) rises. Shortly thereafter, the temperature sense is lost. Hypalgesia is seen shortly thereafter (pin prick) and full anesthesia is reached between 10 and 30 min. Motor paresis follows and is seen to be partial or complete depending on concentration of anesthetic solution. Maximum effect and extent of anesthesia is not reached before 30 min after blocking. Duration largely depends on kind of anesthetic and addition of adrenaline. 2 to 3 (with long-acting drugs 4 to 10) hours are the average.

Segmental Peridural Block

Indications

1. **Diagnostic:** Differential diagnosis of pain in blocked segments.
2. **Therapeutic:** Treating painful states of vasospastic and somatic organic origin, from embolism, traumatism, possibly also thrombophlebitis. To improve circulation and contribute to healing of wounds or operative incisions in conditions where circulation is disturbed; in this respect, it may be used just like a sympatic ganglion block.
3. **Surgical:** No surgical application possible.

Segmental peridural block is especially useful, effective, and indicated in verification of diagnoses or treating visceral diseases such as pancreatitis, colic pains from gall bladder, renal and ureteral disease, Hirschsprung's disease, and similar conditions; please consult table on pages 9–10 for level to be blocked for the respective organ.

Technique

1. **Possibilities:** Always from the dorsal midline between two dorsal spinous processes. Very occasionally also from a paramedial or lateral approach.
2. **Position:** Sitting, prone, or lateral position. In the sitting position, remember that the local anesthetic will tend to move caudally and cause a fall in blood pressure. If the patient is in the sitting or lateral position, the spine should be kept bent, with knees to chest. In the prone position, place pillow(s) under segment to be blocked (chest, abdomen, or pelvis).
3. **Landmarks:** Dorsal spinous processes.
4. **Point of Block:** Segmental nerves, as they traverse the epidural space within the vertebral canal. Unilateral or bilateral block is possible and depends on position of patient; in lateral position, side to be blocked is lower (down).
5. **Procedure:** Between two spinous processes in the dorsal midline, skin is cleansed and (optional) wealed and a peridural needle is introduced perpendicular to the skin in the lumbar levels, while its tip is directed somewhat cranially in thoracic segments. While advancing the needle, attention is paid to the resistance of tissues against the needle. When the resistance is high, the stylett is removed and a 10-ml syringe filled with anesthetic solution is affixed. The plunger of the syringe is now forcefully pushed while advancing the needle extremely slowly, and when the resistance to pressure on the plunger suddenly gives way the needle is arrested; its tip should now rest in the epidural space, into which injecting is very easy. The stream of solution with its pressure pushes the dural sac away, thereby preventing dural puncture. Never aspirate! Now the calculated amount of solution is injected slowly, the needle is withdrawn, and the patient placed in the recumbent (or lateral) position as desired to achieve proper distribution of the anesthetic solution. During the injection care must be taken not to change the position of the needle. In patients that have very thin dura, it may be possible to have the dura pierced by a cough or inadvertant movement of the patient and then spinal anesthesia will result in the respective level; this carries the danger of respiratory and circulatory arrest in higher thoracic segments.

   Note: Epidural injection of a local anesthetic may cause profound drop in blood pressure. It is therefore advised that the necessary drugs be available for application if needed. Blood pressure should be checked frequently shortly after injection and at 5-min intervals later up to 20 to 30 min after block. Cases with such profound drop in blood pressure, however, are much less frequent than with spinal anesthesia.

Evaluation: Check analgesia by pin prick in respective dermatomes.

Complications: Unintended intrathecal injections are not likely to occur if procedure is followed exactly. Only if patient coughs or moves abruptly during injection may this happen.

If palpation of landmarks is not definitely possible as in adipose patients, it is advisable not to carry out any segmental epidural block. For significance of concentration and quantity of solution see respective statement under "caudal block."

Local Anesthetic: 1 to 1.5 ml of any solution per segment, mainly with, but also without adrenaline (1:200,000). If this procedure is done to block sympathetic fibers only, use lowest concentration of anesthetic available.

Onset and Duration: After 3 to 5 min there is subjective and objective rise in skin temperature; shortly thereafter, temperature discrimination is lost. Next hypalgesia appears and 10 to 30 min later full analgesia sets in. Motor paresis of muscles innervated by the respective blocked segments follows and may be partial or complete depending on the concentration of the solution used. Maximum effect never appears before 30 min. Duration between 2.5 and 3 (4 to 10) hr; longer times are achieved only with solutions containing adrenaline, 1:200,000.

Addendum

On p. 78, line 3 from top should be added:

Inadvertent intrathecal injections at higher than midthoracic levels may lead to respiratory and circulatory arrest and will cause unconsciousness and widely dilated pupils. Immediate and proper reanimation for about 6—8 hours will restore normal conditions and leave no sequelae. Epidural segmental injections at such levels therefore should be performed only if reanimation equipment is at hand.

Obturator Nerve Block

Indications

1. **Diagnostic:** For localization of hip pain and evaluation of effect of surgical section of obturator nerve (when planned).
2. **Therapeutic:** Relief of pain in hip joint and of adductor spasm. Pain of hip joint will be influenced in only about 80 percent of cases because 20 percent of joint is innervated by a branch of the ischiadic nerve or by an accessory obturator nerve. Patients with full prosthesis are not helped, however.
3. **Surgical:** None.

Technique

1. **Possibilities:** Only by one approach, from the ventral.
2. **Position:** Supine position, armes crossed behind neck, legs spread.
3. **Landmarks:** Pubic tubercle; point of piercing skin with needle is 1.5 cm laterally and as much caudad of tubercle. Mark skin there.
4. **Point of Block:** Obturator canal.
5. **Procedure:** After shaving (in most patients) of pubic hair and cleansing and wealing (optional) of skin at point of skin mark, an 8- or 10-cm needle is advanced perpendicula to the skin until bone is reached (about 2.5 to 6 cm beneath the skin surface). This is the superior ramus of os pubis and next, needle is withdrawn 2 cm. Change needle direction (see sketch) and advance about 2.5 cm more under minimal contact with bone until tip of needle lies within obturator canal. After aspiration, inject 10 to 15 ml and withdraw needle.

Evaluation: Paresthesias are very rare. Usually, injection is absolutely free of pain, if during advancement of needle minimal amounts of drug are injected. If block is fully effective, there should be loss of force of adduction and external rotation (also crossing of legs!). There may be hypalgesia on a small skin area (see figure: gray area B = skin area, A = analgesia of bone) on medial face of thigh in middle one-third.

Complications: None, if aspiration is done carefully. Otherwise there may be hematomas and intravascular injection. Loss of force of adduction and inward rotation may require that patient be kept under control longer until walking is possible without risk.

Local Anesthetic: 10 to 15 ml, usually without adrenaline.

Onset and Duration: After 5 to 10 min full effect should be reached and last about 1.5 to 3 (4 to 6) hr. It may be mentioned that in several cases of arthrosis of the hip joint, pain-free interval may last very much longer (up to 3/4 or 1 year), requiring another block only then. This, however, cannot be explained.

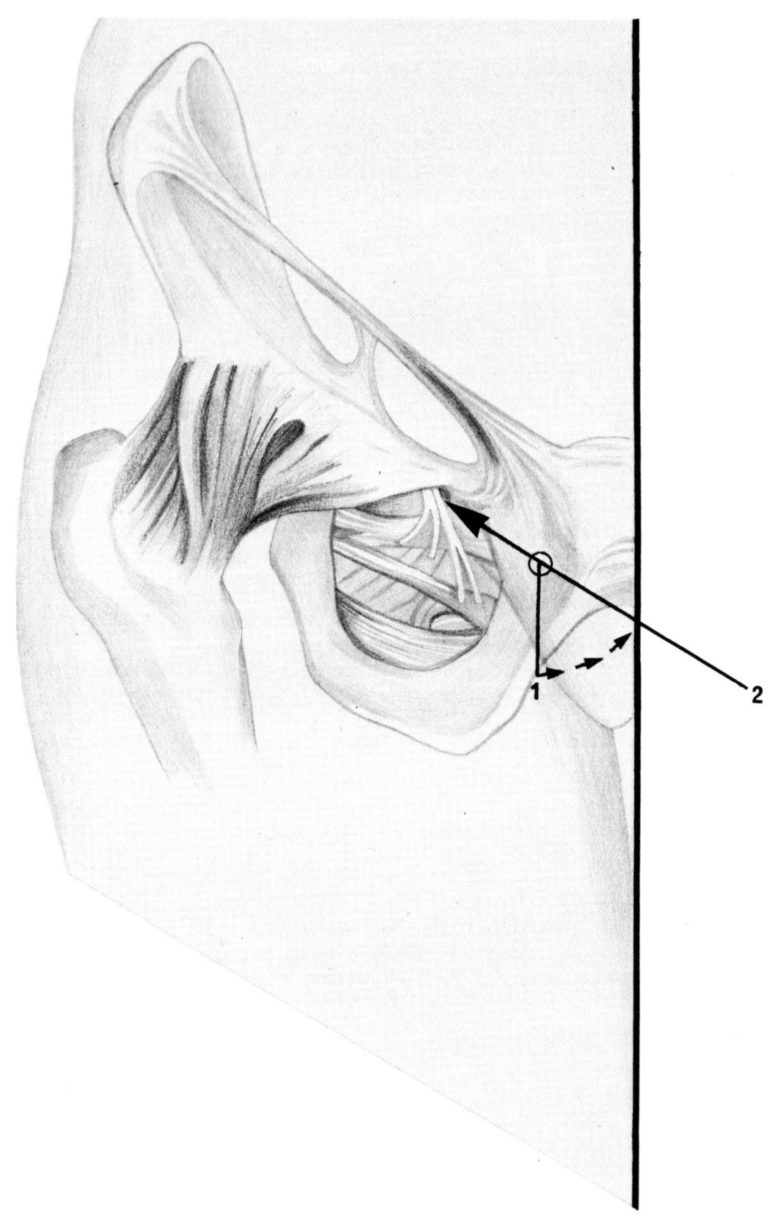

1
2

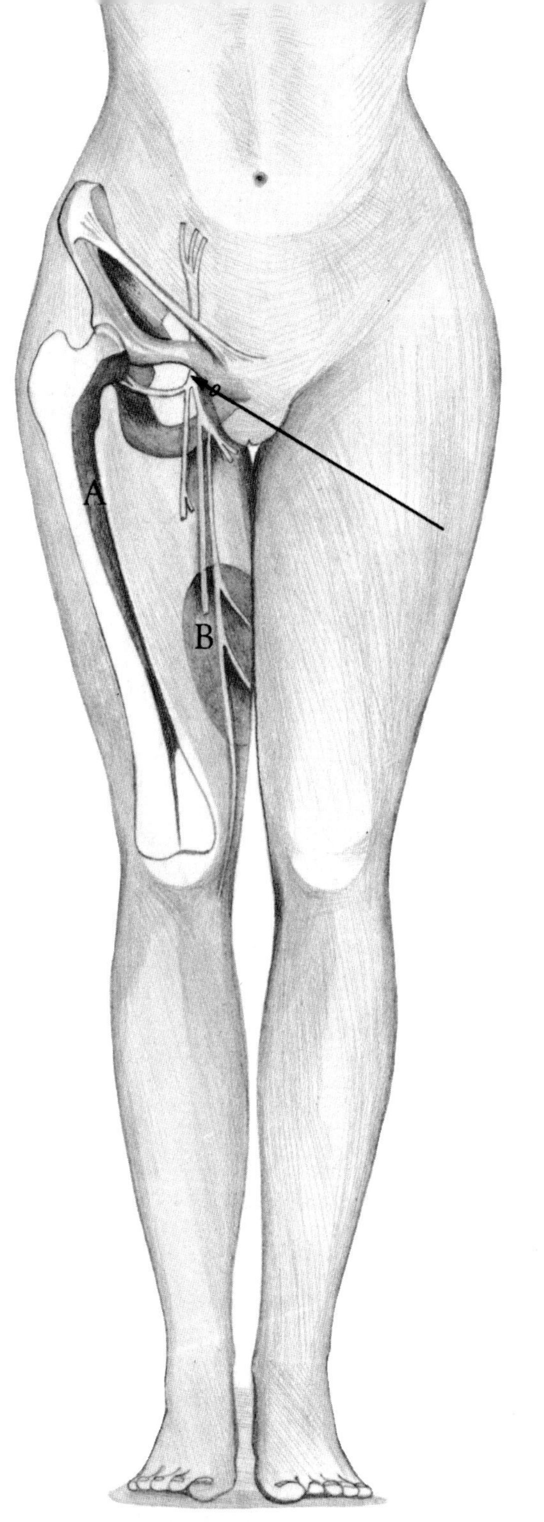
A
B

Ischiadic Nerve Block

Indications

1. **Diagnostic:** Differentiating painful states along course of nerve the block of which is not effective in cases of mechanic root compression.
2. **Therapeutic:** Abolishing pain when origin is peripheral of block. It should be carefully evaluated whether this or another block such as paravertebral somatic, peridural block, or spinal anesthesia will be more effective.
3. **Surgical:** Of no importance (see femoral nerve block).

Technique

1. **Possibilities:** Two transgluteal approaches from dorsal in lateral position of patient and another from dorsal aspect of thigh just caudad of gluteal fold in prone position.
2. Lateral position, side to be blocked up with ipsilateral hip flexed 40° and knee flexed 90° so that long axis of femur will be in line with superior iliac crest. As to rotation, femur should be held in an exactly neutral position.
3. **Landmarks:** According to the technique most frequently used, mark skin over greater trochanter and superior posterior iliac crest. Find half the distance between these two points and place a perpendicular through this midpoint in a caudal-medial direction (see figure on page 84) for about 3 cm. This short line ends at about the point of exit of ischiadic nerve from behind the piriform muscle. Five to six cm distal to this point of injection, another method has its point of injection. Here, the nerve is already much smaller. For this approach, connect skin marks over ischial tuberosity and major trochanter. The point between the caudal and middle third corresponds to the point of injection, under which the ischiadic nerve usually is to be found.
4. **Point of Block:** Ischiadic nerve at its point of exit under the piriform muscle or alternatively at its exit from under the gluteal muscle.
5. **Procedure:** After cleansing and wealing (optional) of skin at point of skin mark, physician sits facing back of patient (who is in lateral position, side to be blocked upwards). Patient is instructed to report paresthesias immediately. A 7- to 10-cm needle is advanced perpendicular to the skin and under slow injection inserted to a depth of about 5 to 8 cm. When paresthesias are reported, arrest needle immediately, aspirate, and inject 5 to 10 ml of local anesthetic. If no paresthesias are elicited and bone is met, it must be the margin of the ileum. Now needle is withdrawn and reinserted in a slightly different direction more medially or laterally. Usually, the nerve is situated about 1 cm toward the skin (from bone). Depth of bone contact therefore is to be noted. Never advance needle to more than 1 cm beyond bone depth. Always try to elicit paresthesias. Should this appear impossible, one may eventually try to infiltratively inject 5 to 20 ml in a fan-like manner and see if an anesthetic effect occurs. However, it is preferable to withdraw the needle and use another approach (see figure on page 85 and paragraph under "landmarks").

   Alternative procedure (carried out on thigh): 2 cm caudad from midpoint of gluteal fold, skin is cleansed and wealed while patient is in prone position. An 8-cm needle is advanced about 5 cm perpendicular to the skin. Paresthesias usually appear at this depth; should this not be the case, withdraw needle and search more laterally or medially to elicit paresthesias. Only then aspirate and inject 5 ml of solution. Because the point of block is somewhat more distally than with the first method, indications for diagnostic or therapeutic block are more limited and do not include cutaneous posterior femoral nerve.

New Method: Patient in supine position, on hard surface, knees supported by small pillow. 3 cm distal to cranial margin of major trochanter, cleanse and weal skin and advance a 10- or 12-cm needle in a transversal plane to a depth of between 6 and 10 cm until paresthesias appear. Now inject 10 ml of anesthetic solution and withdraw needle. For this method, there is no figure.

Evaluation of Effect: Analgesia on back of thigh and leg may be checked by pin prick. Area corresponds to region coarsely dotted in figure on page 88.

Complications: If procedure presented is followed closely there are none. Intravascular injection may happen if aspiration is not done and pelvic organs may be injured if needle is advanced too deep and first method described is used. Therefore watch depth of needle.

Local Anesthetic: 5 to 10 ml of any solution, mainly of higher concentration in therapeutic block, with or without adrenaline, 1:200,000. Never use 96 percent alcohol for this block.

Onset and Duration: 5 to 10 (to 15) min to full effect, which lasts between 2 and 3.5 (to 6 to 14) hr, longer with solutions containing adrenalin.

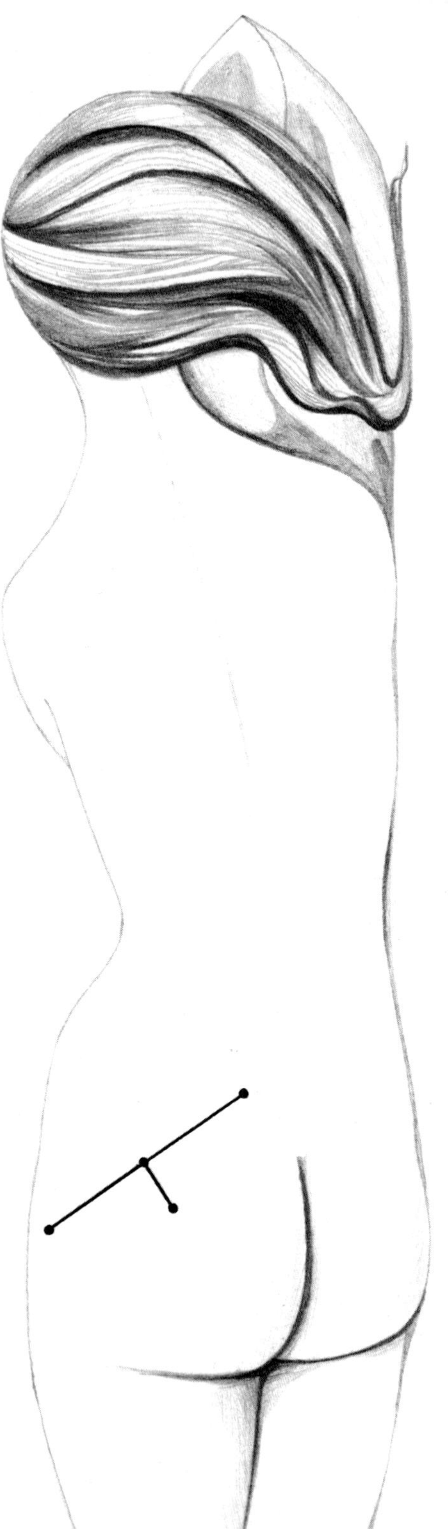

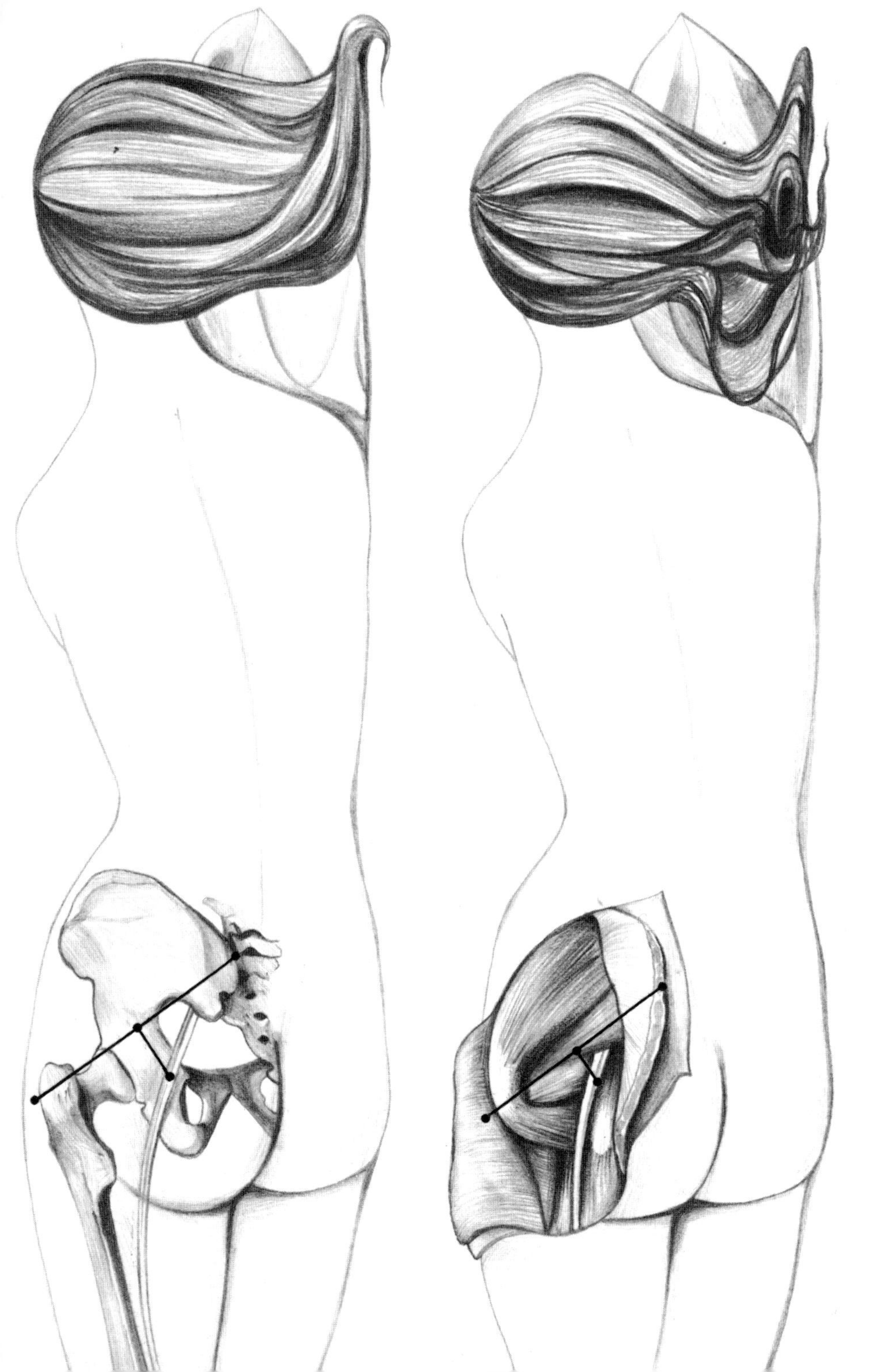

Femoral Nerve Block

Indications:

1. **Diagnostic:** To localize pain in the leg. If pain disappears after this block, the cause of pain is peripheral to the block and root compression does not exist.
2. **Therapeutic:** If pain exists in the peripheral distribution of the nerve, pain may be abolished by this block. The causes are mainly rheumatic disease or muscle spasm of thigh and occur rather infrequently.
3. **Surgical:** None. By combining this block with ischiadic nerve block, some operations on the lower leg are possible.

Technique

1. **Possibilities:** From the ventral.
2. **Position:** Supine position with arms crossed behind neck.
3. **Landmarks:** Palpate femoral artery just caudal of inguinal ligament. Lateral of it the femoral nerve is situated. 1 cm lateral of artery and 1 to 2 cm caudal of inguinal ligament, skin is marked.
4. **Point of Block:** Femoral nerve just beneath skin mark.
5. **Procedure:** After cleansing and wealing (optional) of skin at point of skin mark, the gloved finger of hand not used for injecting palpates femoral artery. It is pulled away medially. A 5-cm needle filled with anesthetic solution on a filled 10- or 20-ml syringe is introduced perpendicular to the skin at the site of the mark and advanced 1.5 to 2.5 cm until its tip is placed next to the femoral artery. The needle tip must be beneath the femoral fascia, which is to be felt as a somewhat greater resistance to puncture. Should paresthesias be elicited the needle is arrested immediately and after aspiration 5 to 10 ml of solution are injected. In case no paresthesias are reported, the solution is spread in a fan-like fashion after aspiration.

Evaluation of Effect: Force of extension of leg and of flexion, abduction and external rotation of thigh is reduced; skin areas on thigh, leg, and foot are found to be analgesic (see small dotted area of figure on page 88) when checked with pin point.

Complications: Intravascular injection is the only complication and should not happen if aspiration is performed correctly.

Local Anesthetic: Without paresthesias, up to 20 ml; with paresthesias, 5 ml of long-acting drug suffice, with or without adrenaline, 1:200,000. Only for diagnostic block use short-acting drug.

Onset and Duration: After 5 to 10 (to 15) min effect should be fully established and should last 2 to 3.5 (5 to 12) hr. The longer durations are achieved with solutions containing adrenaline.

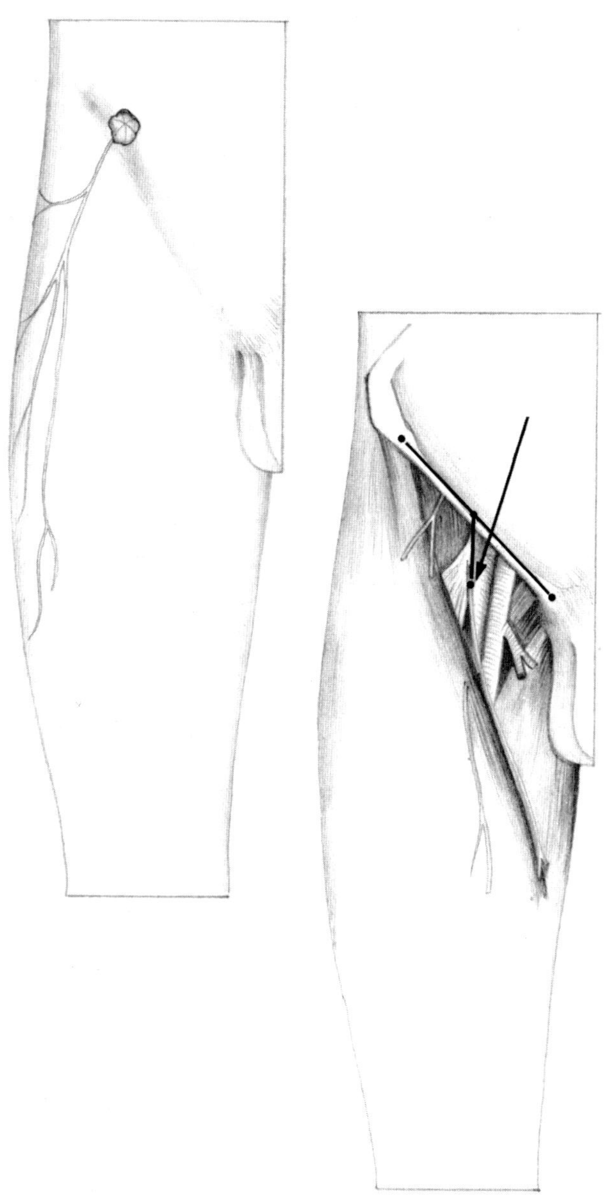

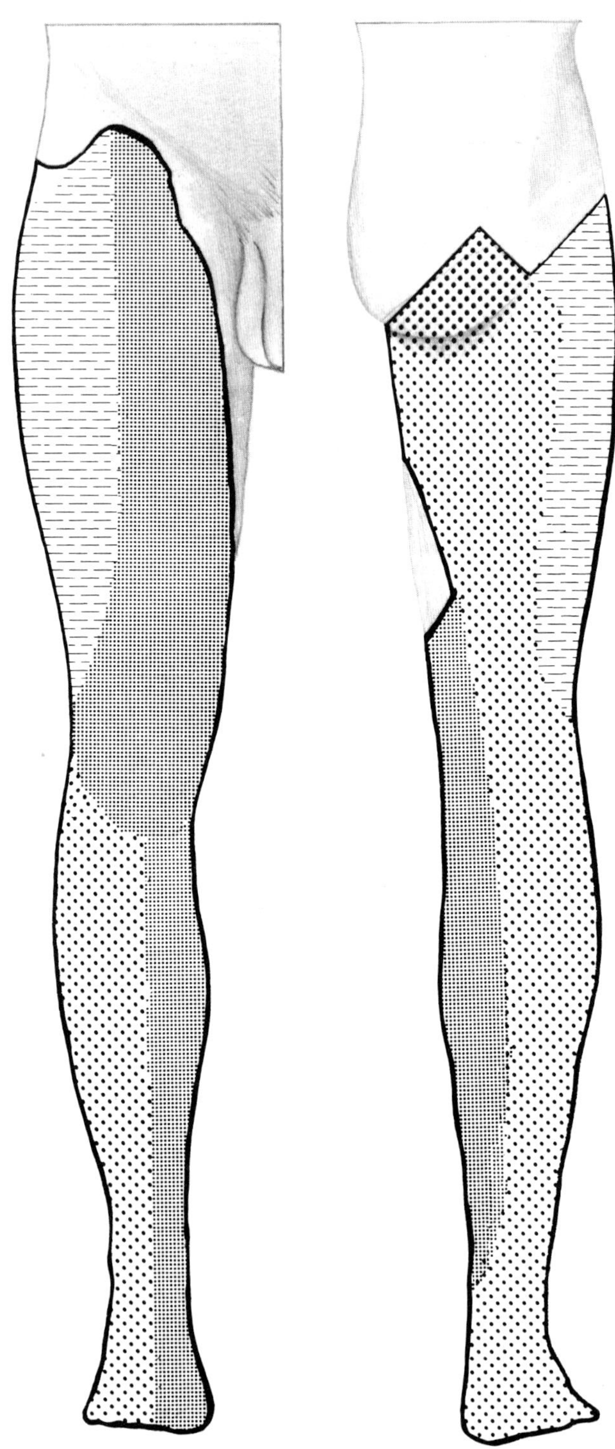

Lateral Cutaneous Femoral Nerve Block

Indications

1. **Diagnostic:** Differentiating pain problems of thigh.
2. **Therapeutic:** Relief of pain in region innervated by nerve (meralgia paresthetica).
3. **Surgical:** None.

Technique

1. **Possibilities:** Percutaneously; or indirectly by paravertebrally blocking the lumbar segmental nerves L2 and 3.
2. **Position:** Supine position, with arms crossed over head.
3. **Landmarks:** Anterior superior iliac crest; 2 to 3 cm medially and just as much caudal of it lies point of injection. Mark skin here.
4. **Point of Block:** Subfascial tissue beneath skin mark where lateral cutaneous femoral nerve should be situated.
5. **Procedure:** After cleansing and wealing (optional) of skin at mark (see figure on page 87), a 5-cm needle on a filled 10-ml syringe is advanced perpendicular to the skin. After reaching fascia and proceeding through it, aspirate and slowly inject depot directly beneath fascia and proceed to bone contact while injecting. Withdraw needle partially, refill syringe, and spread solution in a fan-like manner beneath broad fascia.

Evaluation: Paresthesias are rare. Check sensation with pin point in respective skin segment (see figure on page 88, dashed area).

Complications: None.

Local Anesthetic: 20 ml of short-acting or 10 ml of long-acting drug, with or without adrenaline, 1:200,000.

Onset and Duration: After 2 to 5 (to 10) min effect should be complete and last about 1.25 to 3 (4 to 10) hr.

Block of Supraorbital, Infraorbital, and Mental Nerve

Indications

1. **Diagnostic:** Differentiating trigger zones; testing the possible effectiveness of alcohol injections for trigeminal neuralgia.
2. **Therapeutic:** In the therapy of trigeminal neuralgia when pain is limited to single branch or in case of herpes zoster of one branch. One such injection has to be performed before the decision to use 96 percent alcohol is made.
3. **Surgical:**

Supraorbital nerve	Infraorbital nerve	Mental nerve
None	Dentists rarely use this block for procedures in area of second branch.	None

Technique

1. **Possibilities:** Peripheral branches are reached through the skin. Somewhat more centrally, dentists usually block these nerves from the muscous membranes. Rarely the first branch is blocked at the (posterior) tip of orbita, whereas the second and third branches are reached more centrally in the pterygoid fossa. This possibility is shown separately on pages 93–98.
2. **Position:** Sitting position or reclining without pillow but with small rubber ring under occiput. Patient should not speak, but indicate the incidence of paresthesias by raising one hand.
3. **Landmarks:** See sketch where points of piercing skin and entering bony canals are indicated by open rings or full dots, respectively.
4. **Point of Block:**

Supraorbital nerve	Infraorbital nerve	Mental nerve
Incision of frontal bone on orbital ridge (may be twofold).	Canal in maxilla (direction!)	Canal in mandibula: Please pay attention to direction!

(a) Supraorbital Nerve

5. **Procedure:** After palpating incision in supraorbital ridge, preferably with finger nail, cleanse and weal skin (shaving may be necessary). Perpendicular to skin, perhaps a little from caudally, a 2.5-cm needle is inserted until bone contact is made or paresthesias are reported. 0.5 to 1.0 ml are injected, the needle minimally withdrawn and advanced in a more medial direction to reach the supratrochlear nerve and another 1 ml is injected. Withdraw needle.

Evaluation of Effect: Only paresthesias are relevant.

Complications: None. Sometimes small hematomas may occur (compression).

Remark: Tic douloureux of first branch is extremely rare, is mostly projected from second branch. Therefore, exact exploration is necessary. In cases where pain distribution is in V/1 and V/2, always block V/2 first; should pain in V/1 not be influenced thereby, then block V/1 only.

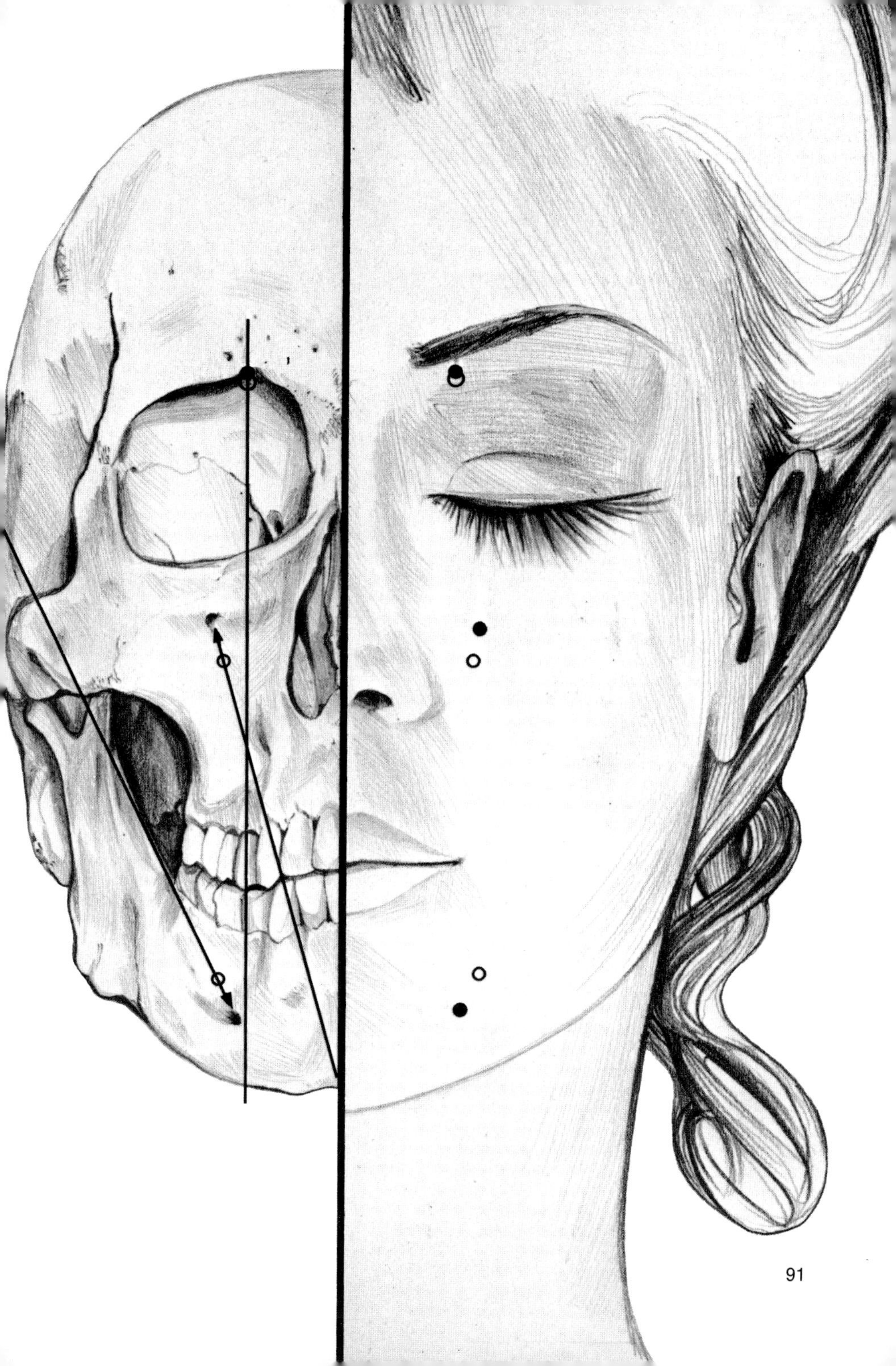

(b) Infraorbital Nerve

5. **Procedure:** After palpation of infraorbital foramen (1.5 to 2 cm lateral of border of nose), mark skin and if only with finger nail. Skin is to be pierced 1 cm caudal and 0.5 cm medial of this mark, where skin is cleansed and wealed (optional). A 4- or 5-cm needle is inserted in a direction pointing cranio-latero-posteriorly, toward the infraorbital foramen. In case of paresthesias arrest needle immediately. Now place a 2-ml syringe onto the needle and inject 1 ml after aspiration. Now needle is advanced slowly into the canal while another 1 ml is being injected. During this, some prefer to rest index finger of left (noninjecting) hand on lower border of orbit just above infraorbital foramen. Now withdraw needle. It may be necessary to press a steril 2 × 2 onto the site of injection for a short while.

Evaluation of Effect: Paresthesias are sought. Testing analgesia using needle tip on cheek, upper lip, including mucous membranes, lower lid, and lateral slope of nose.

Complications: Because the dorsocranial wall of canal may be rather thin, it may happen that bone is perforated and maxillary sinus is punctured when direction of needle is incorrect. Also orbita may be entered. When needle is advanced too far, orbita may also be reached. But temporary double vision is not noteworthy.

(c) Mental Nerve

5. **Procedure:** After palpation of mental foramen (which is about on a line with supraorbital incision and infraorbital foramen), mark this point on skin by imprinting finger nail. Point of piercing skin with needle then is about 0.5 to 1 cm cranio-laterally from there and here, skin is cleansed and wealed (optional). A 4-cm needle is now advanced through this point in a caudal-medial-posterior direction to reach the mental foramen. In case of paresthesias, arrest needle and inject 0.5 to 1.0 ml after aspiration. Advance needle into canal and slowly inject another 0.5 ml. Withdraw needle and (sometimes necessary) press upon site of injection with sterile 2 × 2.

Evaluation of Effect: Paresthesias are sought. Test analgesia by pin prick on lower jaw, lower part of cheek caudal of lip slit, and lower lip including mucous membrane.

Complications: None.

Local Anesthetic: 0.5 to 1.5 ml of any solution, without or with adrenaline. 96 percent alcohol, 0.5 ml.

Onset and Duration: Several minutes after injecting, analgesia sets in; test by pin prick of respective skin area. Lower concentrations of shortacting drugs last only up to 2.5 hr and are apt for diagnostic block whereas long-acting drugs with adrenaline in higher concentrations may last 16 hr and more. If alcohol block is contemplated, wait until block with local anesthetic has lost its effect before injecting alcohol. Sometimes, using long-acting drugs may make alcohol block unnecessary.

Maxillary Nerve Block

Indications

1. **Diagnostic:** Differentiating facial pain.
2. **Therapeutic:** Neuralgia of second branch of trigeminal nerve.
3. **Surgical:** Occasionally in cases of small operations on upper jaw or upper lip and palate in dental surgery.

Technique

1. **Possibilities:** Percutaneously in front of ear (lateral route).
2. **Position:** Supine position, no pillow but small rubber ring under occiput or small roll under neck. Head sould be kept straight and strictly symmetrical, sagittal plane exactly vertical. Note that sketch does not give position of patient.
3. **Landmarks:** Lower margin of zygomatic arch and semicircle of lower mandibula between articular and muscular processus. Just posterior to center of this arch skin mark is placed.
4. **Point of Block:** Maxillary nerve in pterygopalatine fossa.
5. **Procedure:** After cleansing and wealing (optional) of skin at point of skin mark, a 6-cm needle is advanced through the skin at an angle of 45° or less (see sketch) to the horizontal and vertical planes and to the skin as well. The needle just passes by the mandible and holds direction towards the entrance of the optic nerve into the eyeball. Usually the needle meets bone at a depth of about 4 or 5 cm: the pterygoid. Slightly withdrawing the needle and changing direction, the needle slides 0.5 cm past the pterygoid, and now paresthesias should be elicited. After aspiration in three planes the needle is turned so that the bevel shows cranially and 5 ml are injected slowly. The needle is now withdrawn.

Evaluation of Effect: Testing sensibility by pin prick in area of second branch.

Complications: Hemorrhages into cheek or orbit (which take about 2 weeks for resorption) may occur in case a vessel had been punctured. Injection of local anesthetic into the orbit by way of the inferior orbital fissure is of no consequence. Sometimes Horner's syndrome or temporary facial paresis may be observed. Both resolve unattended. While withdrawing needle the anesthetic solution may flow to a branch of the facial nerve or a small amount of air may be injected before the needle is withdrawn, which is to be done routinely when 96 percent alcohol is being used for the block.

Local Anesthetic: 2 to 5 ml of any local anesthetic or 1 ml of alcohol may be used.

Onset and Duration of Effect: 5 (to 15) min after injection effect should be fully established and will last about 1.5 to 3 (8 to 16) hr. Solutions containing adrenaline will reach the longer duration. Alcohol will prolong the effect over several months or longer.

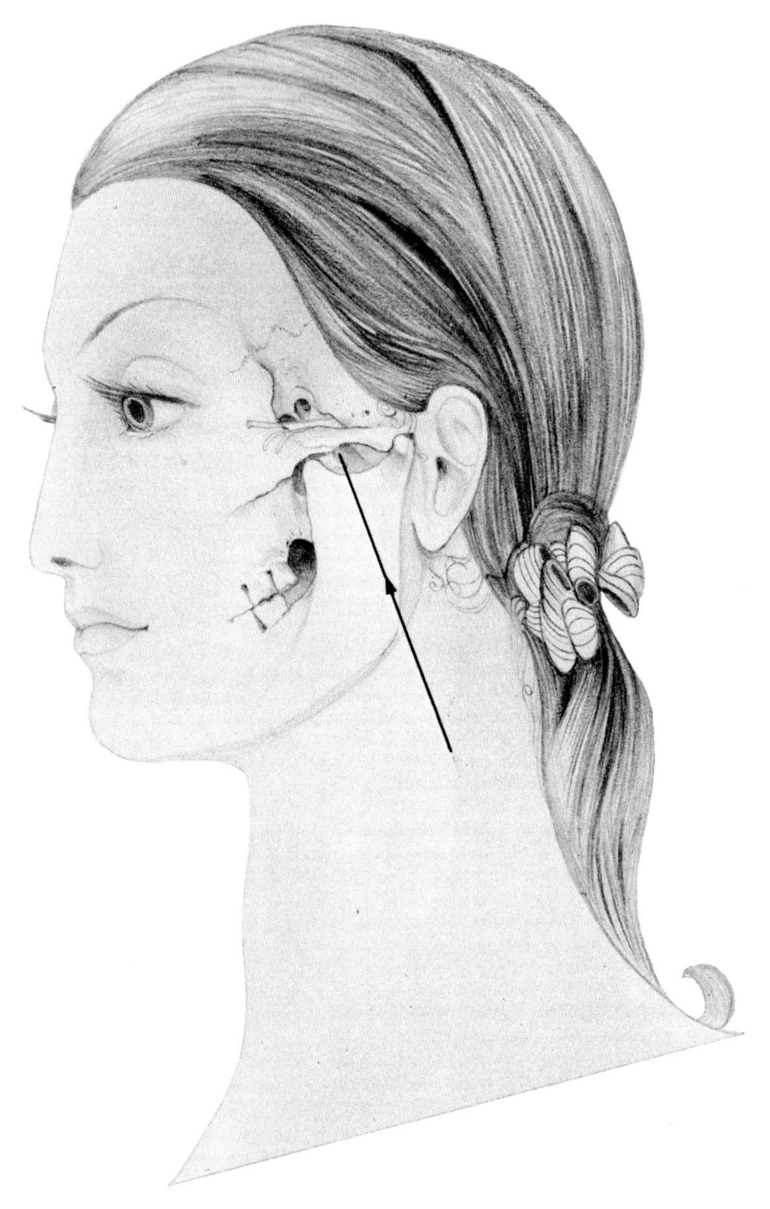

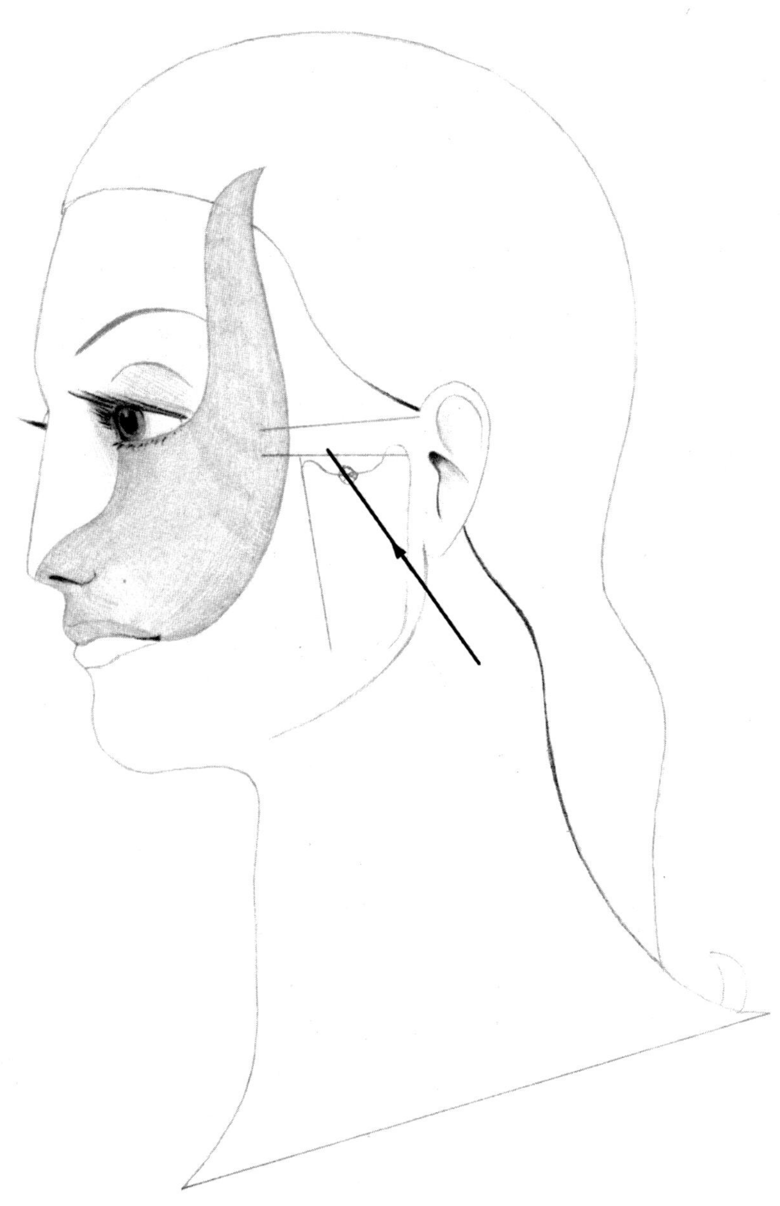

Mandibular Nerve Block

Indications

1. **Diagnostic:** Differential diagnosis of trigeminal (anterior two-thirds of tongue) versus glossopharyngeal (posterior one-third of tongue) neuralgia.
2. **Therapeutic:** Neuralgia of third branch of trigeminal (genuine) or symptomatic neuralgias after tooth extractions, after primary or secondary malignomas of floor of mouth, tongue, or lower jaw; for trismus.
3. **Surgical:** None, except for dental surgical procedures.

Technique

1. **Possibilities:** Percutaneously (= lateral extraoral route); more peripherally also endoorally, the latter only for dental surgical procedures.
2. **Position:** Supine position of patient, no pillow, but small rubber ring under head or small roll under neck.
3. **Landmarks:** Just beneath lower border of zygomatic arch between posterior margin of muscular process and anterior margin of articular process of mandible skin is marked. Usually this is about 1 to 2 cm anterior of tragus.
4. **Point of Block:** Mandibular nerve in pterygopalatine fossa.
5. **Procedure:** After cleansing and wealing (optional) of skin at area of skin mark, a 5 cm needle is introduced through the skin perpendicular to it until paresthesias are elicited. These will be located mainly in the mandible, lower lip, anterior lower incisors, or anterior two–thirds of tongue. If bone is met 4 to 5 cm beneath the skin surface, the tip of the needle is too far anterior and a new insertion is necessary starting subcutaneously. In case of paresthesias arrest needle immediately and withdraw minimally, then aspirate carefully and inject 5 ml of solution of local anesthetic. Withdraw needle under same precautions as mentioned for maxillary block.

Evaluation of Effect: Check sensitivity using pin prick in sensory supply area of this nerve (see figure on page 98).

Complications: Hematoma of cheek may occur following puncture of a vessel. Resorption will take place during 1 to 2 weeks; pressure should be applied locally for a short time. Occasionally, temporary paresis of facial nerve (as in maxillary block) may be seen.

Local Anesthetic: 5 ml of any solution, without or with adrenaline may be used. For longer action 96 percent alcohol is advantageous.

Onset and Duration: 5 (to 15) min after injection anesthesia should be established and last about 1.5 to 3 (8 to 16) hr. Solutions with higher concentration of local anesthetic containing adrenaline reach the longer durations. When using 96 percent alcohol, 0.5 to 1.5 ml suffice to obtain full analgesia after 1 to 5 min which lasts between 3 weeks and 3 months. Pain may be abolished theoretically from 6 months to 3 years but practically the clinically observable effect lasts between 9 and 15 months average.

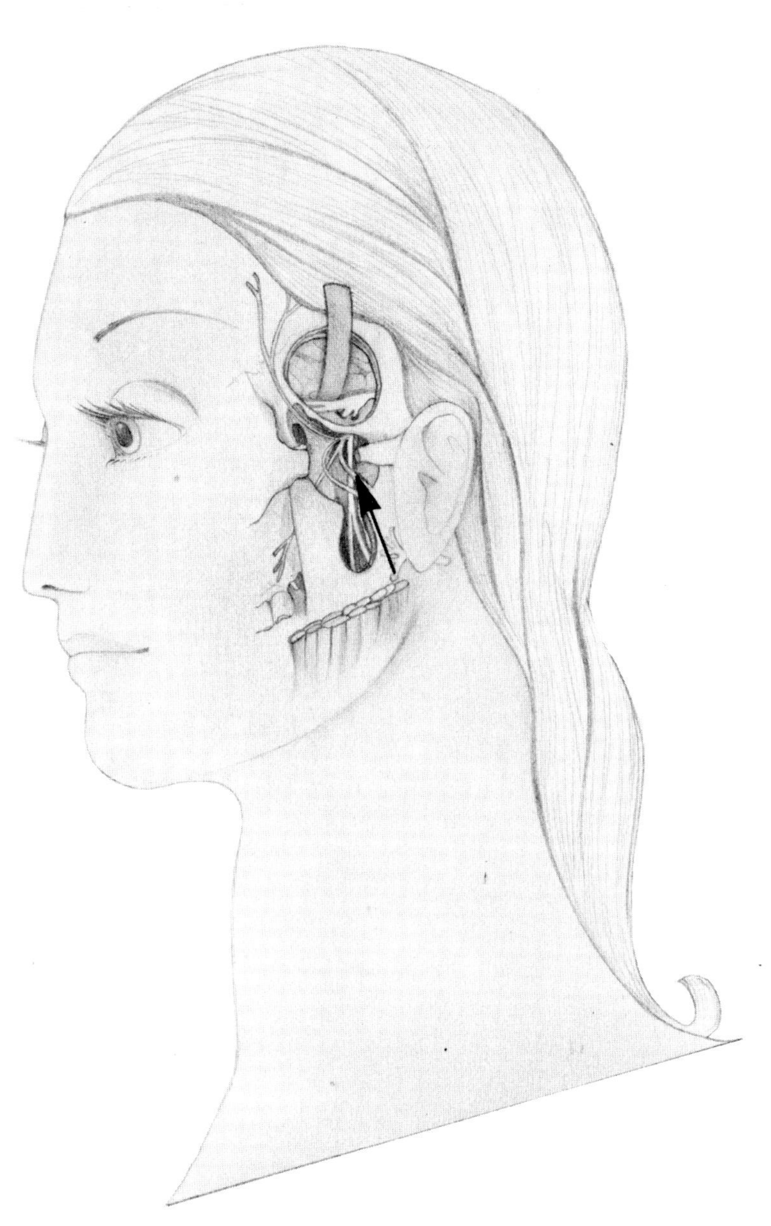

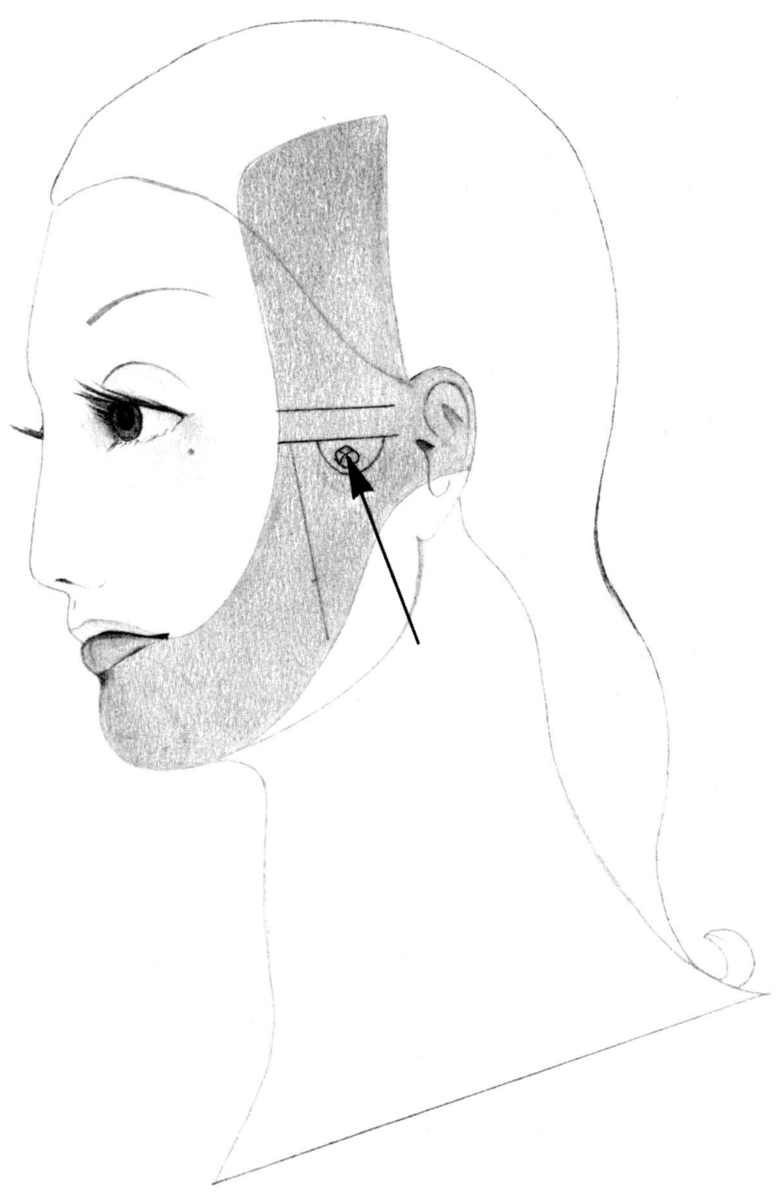

Superior Cervical Ganglion Block

Indications

1. **Diagnostic:** Vasospastic disorders of head, migraine.
2. **Therapeutic:** To obtain vasodilatation of head including cerebral and meningeal vessels. To treat a sensation of a "lump" in throat.
3. **Surgical:** None.

Remark: This block is carried out rather seldom (and then mostly by otolaryngologists) because all effects of this block are also obtained by a stellate block. The close relationship of the injection site to the carotid artery and cranial nerves requires one to limit the amount injected to less than 5 ml.

Anatomy: The superior cervical ganglion is situated along the longus capitis muscle ventral of the transversal processes of the second and third (fourth) cervical vertebrae. It has a close relationship to the loose connective tissue surrounding the internal carotid artery, the jugular vein, and the vagus nerve. The cranial part of the ganglion borders on the hypoglossal, glossopharyngeal, and vagus nerves (laryngic and pharyngic branches of vagus). The ganglion is about 3 to 5 cm long, 6 to 10 mm wide, and 2 to 4 mm thick. It is said to have been formed by fusion of the four uppermost segmental cervical ganglia of the autonomic chain. Its branches reach the internal carotid, jugular vein (also intracranially with its superior branch); the second, third and fourth cervical nerves (lateral branches); pharynx, larynx, and esophagus; thyroid gland; heart (with medial branch, including superior cardiac nerve); common carotid artery and external carotid artery; otic ganglion and submaxillary ganglion (anterior branch); second and third cervical vertebrae and muscles of neck (with posterior branch); as well as an inferior branch to middle cervical ganglion.

Technique

1. **Possibilities:** From the lateral.
2. **Position of Patient:** Supine position, head turned to contralateral side.
3. **Landmarks:** Mastoid process. Mark skin 1 cm caudal and 1 cm medial of this landmark as point of needle entrance.
4. **Point of Block:** Ventral face of longus capitis muscle at level of second cervical vertebra, where superior cervical ganglion is situated.
5. **Procedure:** After cleansing and wealing of skin, a 5-cm needle is advanced through the point of the skin mark in such a way that the tip of the needle makes bone contact with the anterior tubercle of the transverse process of the second cervical vertebra. The bevel should point dorsally. Now mark skin level on needle, withdraw needle to subcutis, and reinsert in same transversal plane but at an angle (to first direction) of 20 to 25° so that the tip of the needle points more anteriorly. Insert 2 cm more and after aspiration (one direction only) up to 5 ml are injected very slowly.

Evaluation of Effect: Horner's syndrome has to appear (miosis, ptosis, and enophthalmus), conjunctival injection, anhidrosis of face and arm of same side, some redness of face, etc. (see under stellate block). Already during injection, observation of pupil will be important.

Complications: Because of anatomical relationship (see above), fast injection or injecting too much anesthetic may lead to vagus block (will lead to tachycardia), pressure on internal carotid artery (temporary cerebral ischemia, vertigo, rarely unconsciousness). Beware of subarachnoidal injection.

Local Anesthetic: Short-acting drugs up to 4 ml, longer-acting drugs should preferably not be used. Never use solutions containing adrenaline.

Onset and Duration: During injection, several minutes after injection at the latest, a Horner's syndrome must appear, or it is to be assumed that the injection site was not correct. Duration: 2 to 3 to 5 hr.

Greater (and Lesser) Occipital Nerve Block

Indications

1. **Diagnostic:** In differentiating occipital headaches and cervical syndrome.
2. **Therapeutic:** For occipital neuralgia.
3. **Surgical:** Together with block of uppermost cervical nerves or cervical plexus, occasionally used for wound excisions or pain from fractures, in former times had been used as anesthesia for operations on cerebellum.

Technique

1. **Possibilities:**
   (a) Superficial site: greater occipital nerve at nuchal line, between onset of trapezius and semispinalis muscles immediately medial of occipital artery (may be palpated very easily). The lesser occipital nerve is situated 2 to 2.5 cm lateral and somewhat caudal of named site.
   (b) Deep site: At exit of greater occipital nerve from under caudal border of inferior oblique head muscle approximately in a transverse plane between atlas and epistropheus, about 3 to 4 cm laterally from sagittal plane.
2. **Position:** Sitting, head slightly bent forward; or in prone position.
3. **Landmarks:** Nuchal line, occipital artery; for block at deep site dorsal spinous processes of uppermost cervical vertebrae.
4. **Point of Block:**
   (a) just medially of occipital artery;
   (b) at turn of greater occipital nerve around caudal margin of inferior oblique head muscle, direction of needle kept to interarcuary slit between atlas and epistropheus.
5. **Prodecure:** After shaving and wealing of skin (usually not necessary) for superficial site, a 5-cm needle on a filled 5-ml syringe is inserted perpendicular to the skin surface to the point of block until paresthesias are elicited. For deep sites, an 8- or 10-cm needle is inserted 3 to 4 cm paramedially in a transversal plane just above the spinous process of the second cervical vertebra also until paresthesias appear. Withdraw needle minimally and, after aspiration, 1 to 2 ml of solution are injected.

Evaluation of Effect: Check pin prick in distribution area of nerve or by disappearance of pain.

Complications: For (a) none; for (b) if needle has been advanced too far, intrathecal injection seems possible.

Local Anesthetic: 1 to 2 ml of any anesthetic, without or with adrenaline; only if no paresthesias are elicited may 3 ml be used.

Onset and Duration of Effect: 3 to 5 (to 10) min after injection full effect should be present and last about 1.5 to 3 (3 to 8) hr using technique for superficial site, at deep site 25 percent less.

Additional Block of Greater Auricular Nerve is not difficult. It should be performed if pain reaches the external auditory canal. This nerve passes from 1.5 to 2 cm caudal of mastoid processus around the posterior margin of the sternocleidomastoid muscle toward the base of the ear. It may be reached at margin of muscle by injecting a small depot (3 to 5 ml) of local anesthetic there. Paresthesias are elicited only rarely.

Remark: Before blocking greater occipital nerve, the cause of neuralgic pain should be sought – as always. If the cause lies in abnormal position of cervical spine or arthritic changes there, relief of pain will be only temporary. Permanent relief is obtained only by removing the cause of pain, e. g., correction of subluxation of cervical vertebra. This block is not difficult to carry out and if used with correct indications very rewarding.

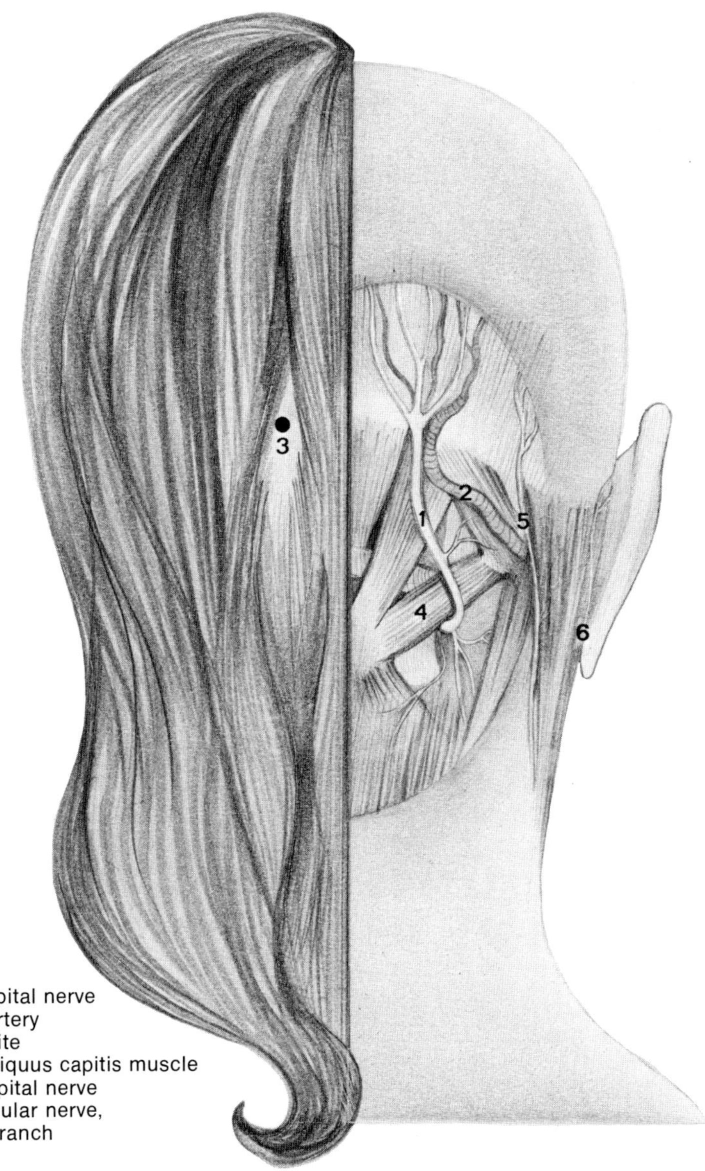

1 Major occipital nerve
2 Occipital artery
3 Puncture site
4 Inferior obliquus capitis muscle
5 Minor occipital nerve
6 Great auricular nerve, posterior branch

Transdermal Stimulation

Introduction

Designated as "transdermal stimulation", the application of an electric current through the skin for purposes of pain relief has recently gained much attention. Actually the various forms of electrotherapy are a domain of physical medicine and rehabilitation. They obtained increasing interest mainly from neurosurgeons since new pain theories were proposed (Melzack and Wall, 1965) and resulted in surgical implantation of peripheral nerve (Meyer and Fields, 1972) or dorsal column (Shealy, 1969) stimulators. The selection of patients for these procedures as an effective means of pain therapy, however, was found to be rather difficult. For purposes of prognosis, stimulation from the skin seemed a proper method of selection. So it was recognized that transdermal stimulation seemed to provide a rationale for pain relief by itself. But pain has no objective criteria by which to judge the effectiveness of a particular current or way of application in a given subject.

Because the effect of an electric current applied from electrodes on the skin must influence nervous elements or structures to relieve pain, an objective proof that such elements are influenced by electric currents must be sought. Pain fibers and sympathetic fibers are of rather similar diameter. Sympathetic fibers have a well-known, definite, and objectifiable influence on the hemodynamics of the region they innervate. Therefore it seemed hopeful to study the influence of transdermally applied currents on cervical sympathetic fibers in the stellate ganglion. The effect observed corresponded absolutely and entirely in direction and extent to the effect a stellate block (conventional procedure, i. e., by injection of a local anesthetic to the ganglion) has on the hemodynamics of brain or upper extremity (Fig. 1). It is not yet clear what mechanisms underlie this action.

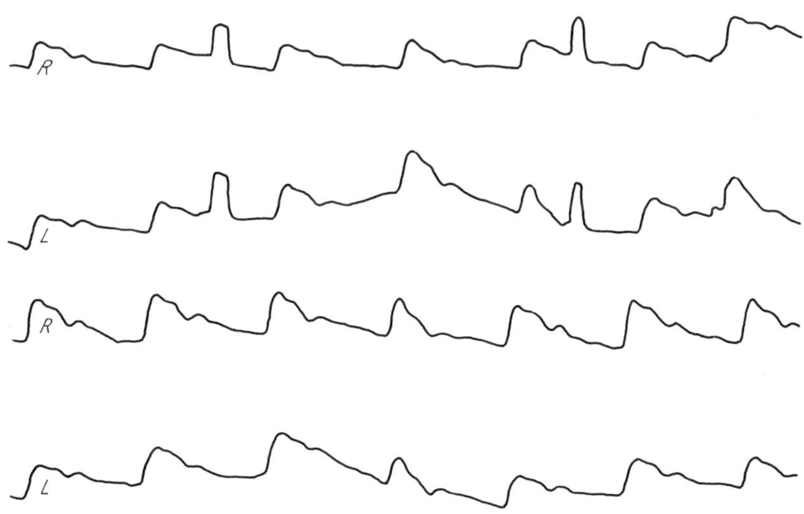

Fig. 1. Pulse wave tracing (arrived at by electric impedance plethysmography or rheography) of right (R) and left (L) arm before (upper two tracings) and 10 min after end of electric stellate block of 20 min duration (applied over right stellate ganglion). Calibration signal equals 0.05 ohms. Paper speed 25 mm/sec. Note higher increase of pulse wave amplitude on side of transdermal electric stimulation

Theories

There have been a number of theories that attempted to explain the clinical observations, but actually none could withstand rigorous control up to now. Therefore it has been decided not to present these theories in detail but to mention them only briefly, in spite of the fact that some of the theories certainly seem interesting to say the least. The interested reader is referred to the original presentations.

Campbell and Taub (1913) think that a peripheral mechanism is responsible for the effect of transdermal stimulation. The theory of Melzack and Wall (1965), surgically transposed by Shealy (1969) and the first one formulated, suggests a spinal mechanism. Most recently Kerr (1975) formulated a theory based on central (cerebral) inhibitory balance phenomena. Kane and Taub (1975) present the history of this not so very new technique of transdermal stimulation.

Even the use of sophisticated examining techniques could not so far elucidate the problem. Computer EEGstudies showed that the evoked potentials (e. g., from an isolated electric stimulus) also reach the cortex after transdermal stimulation; they are not influenced in any way by transdermal stimulation.

Even though it may be assumed correctly that transdermal stimulation does not alter nerve conduction, the term "electric nerve block" has been used to indicate peculiarities of thinking. For practical purposes the reasoning and procedure to be followed are not too different for nerve blocking and transdermal stimulation.

Criteria of Current

That any current is able to decrease pain sensation during its passing through tissue has been known for a long time (Althaus, 1859; Kane and Taub, 1975). But the optimal current should be able to abolish the most severe pain, and the alleviation should last beyond the flow of current for a reasonable length of time. The following facts help to understand why certain criteria will increase the effectiveness of pain relief by an electric current.

1. **Polarity:** Stimulation by direct current causes a soothing, calming effect under the anode (Jantsch and Schuhfried, 1974), whereas under the cathode (the negative pole) there is definite irritation. This would indicate that direct current (also as interrupted direct current, with brief stimulation periods; monophasic current) could have better pain-relieving properties than an alternating (biphasic) current of the same frequency.

2. **Frequency:** It has been known for many decades that application of electric stimuli of varying frequency to a mixed nerve will result in a peculiar phenomenon: higher frequencies (e. g., about 500 cps) will stimulate better and be conducted mainly by larger-diameter (= motor) fibers whereas lower (e. g., 50 cps or less) frequencies will have a better response from the smaller-diameter fibers, e. g., sympathetic or pain fibers. According to findings of Breitbach and Müsch (1938), Gfeller (1929), Schneider (1934), and Valdecas (1935), a current that is expected to influence pain fibers should have a low frequency. Wakim (1953) mentions that stimulation of muscles with low (8 to 32 cps) frequencies leads to vasodilatation. This may be explained by the effect of a current with this low frequency on sympathetic fibers (Fig. 1).

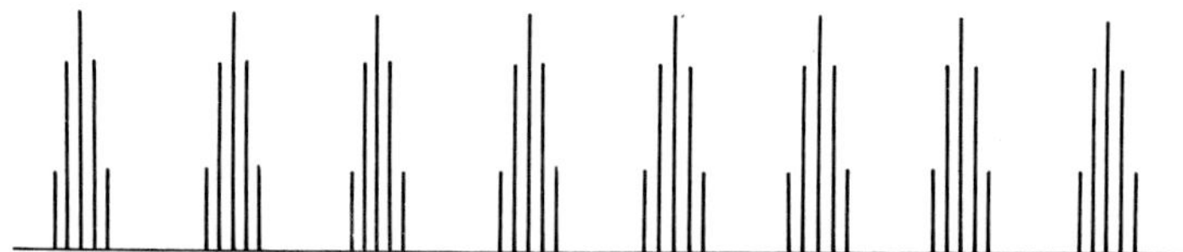

Fig. 2. Diagrammatic presentation of current regarded as optimal so far. (See text)

3. **Duration of Single Stimuli:** The single stimuli should be of a duration that they are not felt by the subject. Here the optimal duration is shorter than 2 msec. Due to this parameter of stimulation it must be stated that application of transdermal stimulation to patients equipped with a cardiac pacemaker is not possible. The pacemaker will sense such a brief stimulus as a fake heart beat and cease stimulating the heart. Only if electrodes are placed far away from pacemaker may it be, that action of pace maker is not influenced. (See figure below.) In such cases ECG monitoring is mandatory.

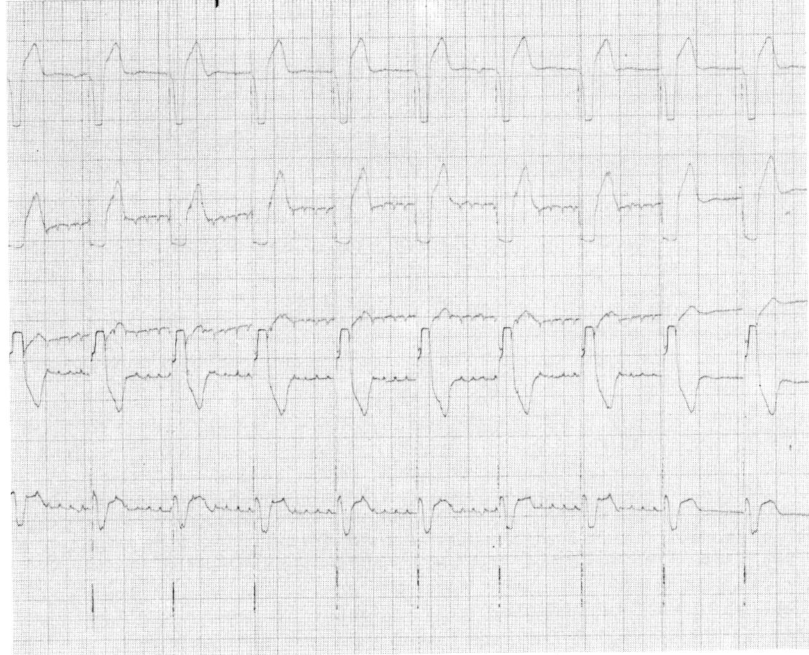

Fig. 3. ECG-monitoring during electric stimulation in a patient with demand pacemaker. Pips of pacemaker downward. Small humps between QRS-complexes, with frequency of about 7 p. sec. are artefacts of stimulation using current shown in Fig. 2

A strong galvanic component of the current was seen to be effective in abolishing pain only when electrodes were applied to painful areas directly, such as in epicondylitis, humeroscapular periarthritis, trochanteric periarthritis, etc. Here also the smaller (different) electrode should be placed over the most painful point and should be the anode. For these cases exponential (galvanic) current may preferably be used.

4. **Electrode Size and Application:** If a nerve is to be influenced electrically, the field through which it passes should be as dense as possible. This makes it imperative that a small electrode be applied over the skin next to the nerve, meaning relatively near to the nerve that is thought to be responsible for the pain one wants to abolish. This is contradictory to all or nearly all electrodes supplied by industry, because all stimulators for transdermal stimulation provide two relatively large elec-

trodes of equal size for both points of application. This small electrode must be anodal and the cathode is connected to a larger (at least six times as large) electrode to keep cathodal stimulation down.
Exact placement of electrodes is critical for best effect and should be determined by a physician only. The suggestion (as made by some manufacturers of stimulators) that "... it is an individual matter of experimentation to search for those areas that seem to work best for your (= the patients) particular pain problems ..." must be rejected. It never leads to optimal results.

Principles of Application

Together with the optimal current, adhering to the following guidelines of application will ensure the best possible results obtainable by present-day technique. One should apply the same method to establish which nerve is responsible for conduction of painful impulses or other noxious impulses that should be interrupted or terminated, just as one does for selecting the nerve or segmental nerve for blocking by injection.

At a site where this nerve is situated closely under the skin the different (smaller, anodal) electrode is placed on the skin. In most instances this will coincide with those points at which a needle is introduced through the skin in executing a nerve block by injection. Therefore, positioning of the patient for transdermal stimulation is the same as for nerve blocks indicated under the respective nerve. There all pertinent indications may also be found together with the landmarks on how to find the site of injection, which is the center of the smaller (anodal) electrode. For influencing the cervical sympathetic (stellate ganglion) or trigeminal nerve a very small different electrode is preferable, which has to be held in place by hand. Its surface is only about 1 cm^2. The other applications mentioned will require a surface area of about 2.5×2.5 cm (1×1 in) as an anodal electrode. The indifferent electrode should measure about six times the area of the anodal electrode and be placed about opposite on the surface of the body or over areas mentioned under special guidelines. The smallest electrode (hand electrode, for use on stellate ganglion, etc.) is a metal semiglobe on a handle. For this electrode paste should be used. As a different electrode, conductive silicone rubber is used and the use of paste is optional even though advisable. The large indifferent electrode might be either a flexible lead sheet plate within a moistened foam rubber envelope (interchangeable) or again a conductive silicone rubber. For fixation of electrodes rubber bands are preferred.

In the beginning, stimulation is done once a day, preferably at time just prior to expected maximum of pain sensation. After relief is obtained, once a week may suffice and after 3 or 4 such intervals several weeks to months may be free of pain depending on case. On first indication of recurring pain, resume stimulations at daily intervals for a few times.

Each stimulation session should be carried over 20 min, the strength of the current being readjusted about every 5 min to a level that is sensed as a strong but not unpleasant event. In some cases the first application will result in improvement of the condition but in most instances a series of five treatments has proven advisable for lasting effect. More applications are necessary in cases of severe pain of malignant origin. But in these desperate cases the use of opiates may be postponed for a considerable length of time or often even obviated. The average rate of success in treatment with this technique has been seen to be over 60 percent if all the various indications are included.

to individual transdermal electric stimulation of nerves (electric nerve blocks)

Stellate Ganglion

A very small electrode, about 1 cm^2, is preferably held by hand to the skin site where a needle would penetrate the skin if a block by injection were made. This must be the anode. The cathode is placed on the skin overlying the scapula of the same side. Any such application, for 20 min, equals a stellate block by injection in its effect, at least on hemodynamics of brain and arm. See the figure on page 105. Indications are the same as for stellate block (vide there). In spite of this, no blood pressure drop has been observed so far and no other side effects occur. Extremely long-lasting results have been seen in the treatment of hyperhidrosis of the upper half of the body. Correct electrode placement always will lead to Horner's syndrome and sometimes to disturbance of function of recurrent nerve (= coarse voice for a few hours).

Lumbar Sympathetic Block

7 to 9 cm paravertebrally at the level of the third lumbar nerve is located the center of the different electrode (anode). The size of the electrode should be 1 × 1 in. The cathode should be opposite on abdominal wall at the same level about midline position. Indications are as for lumbar sympathetic block. Very good results have been seen in cases of circulatory disturbances of the legs. Hyperhidrosis of the lower half of body also responds very well.

Deep Cervical Plexus

Because this plexus lies close under the skin, it may be reached easily and successfully by electric stimulation from the skin. The description of pain by a patient will indicate which nerve is involved and the skin over the respective transverse process (in a position of the patient corresponding to the one given for block of this plexus by injection) is the site for applying the anodal current. Cathode is placed either in back over the seventh cervical and first to third thoracic dorsal spinous processes or around the upper arm over the medial bicipital fold. Most important indications are pain by impingement of metastatic malignant lesions secondary to carcinoma of the breast or bronchial carcinoma pressing on or invading the respective nerve, or through toxic neuropathy.

Brachial Plexus

The same directions given for deep cervical plexus also hold for this plexus and its nerves. Electrode size, placement, and indications are identical, as for block by injection.

Thoracic Nerves

Placement of the electrode is such that the center of the small different anodal electrode overlies the site at which the needle (of a block by injection) penetrates skin. This is true for paravertebral, posterior axillary, or other placement. The cathode is placed on the opposite part of the body or at a distance along the respective intercostal nerve. Indications are, e. g., herpes zoster neuralgia, metastatic involvement of intercostal nerve or of rib. In herpetic neuralgia, five to ten applications suffice in most cases, whereas in malignant pain, two applications a day might initially be necessary and after 2 or 3 weeks larger intervals are possible.

Lumbar Segmental Nerves

Placement of electrodes follows the suggestions given above. The different electrode is placed with its center over the site where the needle pierces the skin for injection block. The indifferent electrode is placed on the ipsilateral side on the abdominal wall between the midline and the iliac crest. Indications are lumbar segmental pain, and after lumbar disk operations with residual pain or toxic neuralgia; malignant lesions involving lumbar segments usually are multisegmental and not very suitable for transdermal stimulation. However, if only one nerve is involved, fair results have been obtained and a trial is worthwhile because it may be possible to circumvent injections of narcotics by it.

Sacral Nerves

In principle, what has been said about lumbar nerves applies also for sacral segments, especially as far as malignant pain is concerned. If pain from a recurrent rectal malignancy is strictly one-segmental in its distribution, very rewarding results have been seen. But the clear description of pain by the patient is a prerequisite *sine qua non.*

Obturator Nerve

The indications for block by local anesthetics is the same for this "electric block." Good results have been obtained by placement of the cathode over the ipsilateral buttock and the anode over the site of the skin mark mentioned under the identical block by injection. Hip joint pain is usually relieved after five to ten sessions of 20 min each. But it should be recalled that metal within the body (also prostheses) is a contraindication for the application of electric current to this area. Also, unfortunately, a block by injection does not give relief to total joint prostheses.

Ischiadic Nerve

Different electrode placement is best over the gluteal fold, at the site of needle insertion if no segmental pain is described by the patient (then segmental lumbar application is preferable). The cathode is best placed over the ventral aspect of the thigh just under the inguinal ligament, or alternatively over the dorsal aspect of the thigh at its mid-third.

Trigeminal Nerve

The electrode position is the anode as a hand electrode (see stellate ganglion) at the site of needle entrance for block of maxillary or mandibular nerve block for its injection in pterygopalatine fossa and cathode (1 in^2 size) over the peripheral exit of the affected branch. Only genuine neuralgia responds well; symptomatic neuralgia such as after dental surgery gives rather poor results. In the former, five to ten sessions give about 50 percent relief. Pain caused by malignancies also responds well.

References

(a) Nerve Blocks

1 **Auberger, H. G.:** Praktische Lokalanaesthesie. G. Thieme, Stuttgart, 1969.

2 **Auberger, H. G.:** Regionale Schmerztherapie. G. Thieme, Stuttgart, 1971.

3 **Beck, L., and H. Stockhausen:** Die transvaginale Pudendus-Anaesthesie mit Hilfe neuer Spezialnadeln. Geburtshilfe und Frauenheilkunde. G. Thieme, Stuttgart, **26:** 932–937, 1966.

4 **Bonica, J. J.:** The Management of Pain. Lea and Febiger, Philadelphia, 1954.

5 **Braun, N.:** Die Lokalanaesthesie, ihre wissenschaftlichen Grundlagen und praktische Anwendung. J. A. Barth, Leipzig, 1905.

6 **Buck-Gramcko, D., and J. Geldmacher:** Leitungsanaesthesie in der Handchirurgie. Der Chirurg, Springer-Verlag, **36:** 513–516, 1965.

7 **Dietrich, H. H.:** Die Bedeutung der Lokalanaesthesie für das kleinere Krankenhaus. Die Medizinische Welt, F. K. Schattauer, Stuttgart, **49:** 2751–2753, 1965.

8 **Eccles, J. C.:** The Neurophysiological Basis of Mind. The Clarendon Press, Oxford, 1953.

9 **Eccles, J. C.:** The Physiology of Nerve Cells. The Johns Hopkins Press, Baltimore, 1957.

10 **Eichholtz, F.:** Lehrbuch der Pharmakologie, 6. Aufl., Springer, Berlin, Göttingen, Heidelberg, 1948.

11 **Eriksson, E.:** Atlas der Lokalanaesthesie. (Deutsche Übersetzung des schwedischen Originales, Munksgard, Kopenhagen, 1969.) G. Thieme, Stuttgart, 1970.

12 **Frodermann, H. and J. Hagelstein:** Über die Bedeutung der Leitungs- und Lokalanaesthesie im Unfallkrankenhaus. Der Krankenhausarzt **38:** 1–12, 1965.

13 **Fuchsig, P.:** Technik und Resultate der Unterbrechung des lumbalen Grenzstranges mit Alkoholinjektionen. Wien. med. Wschr. **98:** 201–205, 1948.

14 **Goodman, L. S., and A. Gilman:** The Pharmacological Basis of Therapeutics. The Macmillan Company, New York, 1970.

15 **Grimmeisen, H.:** Die Bedeutung der Lumbalanaesthesie bei operativ-orthopädischen Eingriffen. Der Krankenhausarzt, G. Braun, Karlsruhe, **39:** 1–16, 1966.

16 **Grünberger, V., E. Reinold, and P. Wagenbichler:** Geburtsanaesthesie durch Parazervikalblockade. Wiener klinische Wochenschrift **81:** 747–749, 1969.

17 **Gunther, R., and J. Bauman:** Obstetrical caudal anesthesia. Anesthesiology **31:** 5, 1969.

18 **Haas, E.:** Lokalanaesthesie – mit oder ohne Adrenalin. Laryngologie – Rhinologie – Otologie, **45:** 274–279, 1966.

19 **Harley, N., and J. Gjessing:** A critical assessment of supraclavicular brachial plexus block. Anaesthesia **24:** 564, 1969.

20 **Jost, A.:** Lokalanaesthesie in der Ambulanz und im Operationssaal. Fortschritte der Medizin **82:** 27–29, 1964.

21 **Kilian, H.:** Lokalanaesthesie und Lokalanaesthetika. G. Thieme, Stuttgart, 1973.

22 **Krause, W.:** Das lumbale Wurzelreizsyndrom und die paravertebrale Blockade nach Reischauer. Zeitschrift für Orthopädie und ihre Grenzgebiete **102:** 236–243, 1966.

23 **Krebs, A.**: Geburtshilfliche und gynäkologische Operationen in Lokalanaesthesie. Die Therapie-Woche **17:** 754, 1967.

24 **Krieger, K.**: Ein Erfahrungsbericht aus der Plastisch-kosmetischen- und Venenchirurgie unter besonderer Berücksichtigung der Lokalanaesthesie. Die Medizinische Welt **33:** 1735–1738, 1964.

25 **Kulenkampff, D.**: Die Anaesthesierung des Plexus brachialis, Dtsch. med. Wschr. **38:** 1878–1880, 1912.

26 **Macintosh, R. R. and W. W. Mushin:** Örtliche Betäubung, Plexus brachialis, Springer-Verlag, Berlin–Heidelberg–New York, 1967.

27 **Matthes, H.**: Untersuchungen und Ergebnisse bei der supraclaviculären Blockade des Plexus brachialis. Der Anaesthesist **14:** 107–109, 1965.

28 **Matthes, H. and P. Schabert:** Regionale Analgesie im Bereich der oberen Extremität. Praktische Anaesthesie und Wiederbelebung **3:** 9–16, 1968.

29 **Moore, D. C.**: Complications of Regional Anesthesia. C C Thomas, Springfield, Ill., 1955.

30 **Moore, D. C.**: Regional Block. C C Thomas, Springfield, Ill., 1969.

31 **Murphy, P. J., et al.**: Assessment of paracervical nerve block anesthesia during labour. Brit. med. J. **1:** 526, 1970.

32 **Nahor, A., J. Milliken, R. Minton, and J. Fine:** Technique of Celiac Blockade for Relief of Splanchnic Ischemia. J. Amer. Med. Assoc. **192:** 600–602, 1965.

33 **Nolte, H.**: Einzeitige doppelseitige Stellatumblockade in der Therapie der Lungenembolie. Der Anaesthesist **13:** 160–163, 1964.

34 **Nolte, H.**: Die Technik der Lokalanaesthesie. (In der Reihe Anaesthesie und Wiederbelebung.) Springer-Verlag, Berlin–Heidelberg–New York, 1966.

35 **Nolte, H. and J. Meyer:** Regionale Anaesthesie mit dem Langzeitanaesthetikum Bupivacain. Internationales Symposium, G. Thieme, Stuttgart, 1971.

36 **Patrick, J.**: The Technique of Brachial Plexus Anesthesia. Brit. J. Surg. **27:** 734–739, 1940.

37 **Ritchie, J. M., P. J. Cohen, and R. D. Dripps:** Local Anesthetics. In: Goodman, L. S., and A. Gilman: The Pharmacological Basis of Therapeutics. The Macmillan Company, New York, 1970.

38 **Schmidt, R. F.**: Neurophysiologie. Springer-Verlag, Berlin–Heidelberg–New York, 1971.

39 **Solonen, K. A., and L. Tarkanen:** Die intravenöse Anaesthesie in der Handchirurgie. Archiv für orthopädische und Unfallchirurgie, **60:** 115–121, 1966.

40 **Steenberge, A. L. van:** L'anesthésie péridurale. Masson & Cie, Paris, 1969.

41 **Stockhausen, H.**: Über die Anwendung des paracervicalen Blocks zur Geburtserleichterung. Geburtshilfe und Frauenheilkunde **27:** 266–270, 1970.

42 **Titze, A.**: Die Leitungsanaesthesie in der Handchirurgie. Ihre Vor- und Nachteile. Chir. Praxis **6:** 165–170, 1962.

43 **Telivuo, L., and R. Katz:** The effects of modern intravenous local analgesics on respiration during partial neuromuscular block in man. Anesthesia **25:** 30, 1970.

44 **Vacek, V., and L. Puzanova:** Umspritzung des Plexus coeliacus beim septischen Schock. Med. Klinik **61:** 1297–1298, 1966.

45 **Winkler, R.**: Erfahrungen bei Routineoperationen unter Lokalanaesthesie in einer HNO-Abteilung. Die Therapiewoche **14:** 9, 481, 1964.

(b) Transdermal Stimulation

1 **Althaus, J.:** Über elektrische und elektrochemische Anaesthesie. Wiener med. Wschr. 9: 433–435, 1859.

2 **Breitbach, A., and H. Müsch:** Selektive Reizung vegetativer Nervenfasern im Nervus ischiadicus des Frosches. Pflügers Arch. f. d. ges. Physiol. **241:** 360–369, 1938.

3 **Campbell, J. N., and A. Taub:** Local Analgesia from Percutaneous Electrical Stimulation. A Peripheral Mechanism. Arch. Neurol. (Chicago) **28:** 347–350, 1973.

4 **Gfeller, F.:** Untersuchungen über die allgemeinen physiologischen Eigenschaften des Sympathicus geprüft am Nervus accelerans des Frosches. Z. Biol. **89:** 202–216, 1929.

5 **Jantsch, H., and F. Schuhfried:** Niederfrequente Ströme zur Diagnostik und Therapie. W. Maudrich, Wien–München–Bern, 1974.

6 **Jenkner, F. L.:** Möglichkeiten und Besonderheiten chirurgischer Schmerzausschaltung. Acta Chir. Austr. **5:** 123–129, 1973.

7 **Kane, K., and A. Taub:** A History of Local Electrical Analgesia. Pain **1:** 125–138, 1975.

8 **Kerr, F. W. L.:** Pain. A Central Inhibitory Balance Theory. Mayo Clin. Proc. **50:** 685–690, 1975.

9 **Melzack, R., and P. D. Wall:** Pain Mechanisms: A New Theory. Science **150:** 971–979, 1965.

10 **Meyer, G. A., and H. L. Fields:** Causalgia Treated by Selective Large Fiber Stimulation of Peripheral Nerve. Brain **95:** 163–168, 1972.

11 **Nashold, B. S., and H. Friedman:** Dorsal Column Stimulation for Control of Pain. J. Neurosurg. **36:** 590–597, 1972.

12 **Ray, C. D.:** Control of Pain by Electrical Stimulation. A Clinical Follow-up Review. Advances in Neurosurg. **3:** 216–224, 1975.

13 **Schneider, D.:** Über die vasomotorische Benervung der Extremitäten. Naunyn-Schmiedebergs Arch. **176:** 111–140, 1934.

14 **Sheally, C. N., N. Tashlitz, J. T. Mortimer, and D. Becker:** Electrical Inhibition of Pain: Experimental Evaluation. Anesth. and Analg. Current Research **46:** 299–305, 1966.

15 **Shealy, C. N.:** Dorsal Column Electrohypalgesia. Headache **9:** 99–108, 1969.

16 **Valdecas, F. G.:** Die Physiologie der Skelett-Muskel-Durchblutung. Z. Biol. **96:** 28–34, 1935.

17 **Wakim, K. G.:** Influence of Frequency of Muscle Stimulation on Circulation on the Stimulated Extremity. Arch. Phys. med. **34:** 521–1953.

SUBJECT INDEX